OSHA
Guidebook for Labs

SECOND EDITION

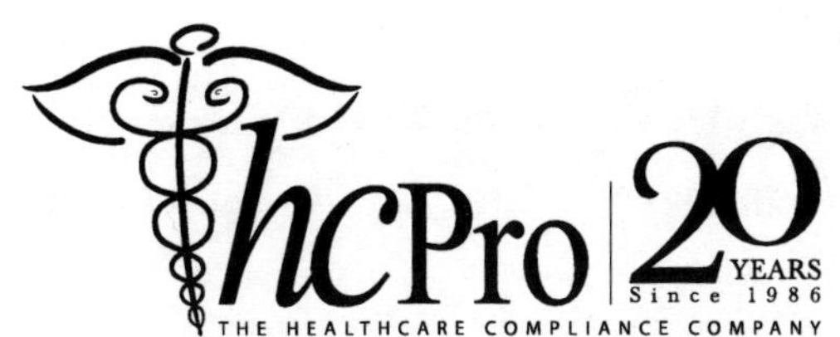

OSHA Guidebook for Labs, Second Edition is published by HCPro, Inc.

 5 4 3 2 1

ISBN 1-57839-889-4

HCPro, Inc., provides information resources for the healthcare industry.

Terry Jo Gile, Reviewer
Mike Mirabello, Senior Graphic Artist
Jean St. Pierre, Director of Operations
Shane Katz, Cover Designer
Bob Croce, Group Publisher

Arrangements can be made for quantity discounts. For more information, contact:

HCPro, Inc.
P.O. Box 1168
Marblehead, MA 01945
Telephone: 800/650-6787 or 781/639-1872
Fax: 781/639-2982
E-mail: *customerservice@hcpro.com*

Visit HCPro at its World Wide Web sites:
www.hcpro.com* and *www.hcmarketplace.com

09/2006
20965

Contents

Introduction . . . v

Acronyms and abbreviations . . . vi

Access to records (1904, 1910, 1020, 1913.10, and others) . . . 1

Air contaminants (1910.1000) . . . 5

Asbestos (1910.1001 for general industry and 1926.1101 for construction) . . . 11

Bloodborne pathogens (1910.1030) . . . 45

Compressed gases (1910.169) . . . 67

Confined spaces (1910.146) . . . 73

Construction/renovation (1926) . . . 87

Electrical safety (1910, subpart S) . . . 101

Emergency plans (1910.38) . . . 105

Emergency response/HAZWOPER (1910.120) . . . 107

Employee health services . . . 115

Ergonomics (voluntary guideline) . . . 125

Ethylene oxide (1910.1047) . . . 131

Exiting (1910.36) . . . 149

Eye/face protection (1910.133 and various standards) . . . 151

Eyewash/emergency shower (1910.151) . . . 153

Fire prevention and protection (1910.155 to 1910.165) . . . 155

Formaldehyde (1910.1048) . . . 169

General duty clause . . . 189

Glutaraldehyde . . . 191

Hazard communication standard (29 CFR 1910.1200) . . . 195

Hearing/noise exposure (1910.95) . . . 209

Laboratory standards (1910.1450) . . . 219

Lasers (guidance) 237
Laundry/housekeeping 251
Lead (1926.62 [construction work] and 1910.1025 [general industry]) 263
Lockout/tagout (1910.147) 277
Machine guarding (1910.212) 287
Medical first aid (1910.151) 289
Mercury 291
Personal protective equipment (1910.132) 295
Radiation (1910.1096 [ionizing] and 1910.97 [non-ionizing]) 303
Recordkeeping (1904) 315
Respiratory protection (1910.134) 335
Welding (1910.254 and 252) 357
Workplace violence (voluntary guideline) 359
Xylene 365
Appendix A: State occupational safety health plans 373
Appendix B: OSHA standards training frequency 385

Introduction

This reference guide reviews the top Occupational Safety and Health Administration (OSHA) standards with which laboratory safety managers regularly deal. Although no chapter is intended to be a substitute for an entire standard, this book outlines the major points of the laboratory-related regulations in an easy-to-read format. You will be able to navigate through the requirements quickly and confidently.

We've packed a lot of vital information into this guide. But, knowing how busy you are, we have kept it manageable and practical. All topics are organized alphabetically, and each page is marked with a shaded tab, enabling you to flip quickly through the guide to find the information you need. Also, commonly used acronyms and abbreviations are listed at the start of the guide for handy reference.

It is our job to review the information and condense it into an understandable guide so that you can have everything related to OSHA and laboratories in one place. We hope you find it indispensable.

Acronyms and abbreviations

ACGIH: American Conference of Governmental Industrial Hygienists

ACIP: Advisory Committee on Immunization Practices

ACM: asbestos-containing materials

ANSI: American National Standards Institute

ASME: American Society of Mechanical Engineers

BLS: Bureau of Labor Statistics

BSI: body substance isolation

CAT: computerized axial tomography

CERCLA: Comprehensive Environmental Response, Compensation, and Liability Act

CGA: Compressed Gas Association

CDC: Centers for Disease Control and Prevention

CHO: chemical hygiene officer

CHP: chemical hygiene plan

CPR: cardiopulmonary resuscitation

dBA: decibels on the A scale

DOT: Department of Transportation

EAP: employee assistance program

EC: environment of care

EHS: employee health service

EMS: emergency medical service

EPA: Environmental Protection Agency

EPCRA: Emergency Planning and Community Right-to-Know Act

ESLI: end-of-service-life indicator

EtO: ethylene oxide

FDA: Food and Drug Administration

FPM: feet per minute

HAZWOPER: Hazardous Waste Operations and Emergency Response

HBV: hepatitis B virus

HEPA: high-efficiency particulate air

HICPAC: Hospital Infection Control Practices Advisory Committee

HIV: human immunodeficiency virus

Hz: hertz

IARC: International Agency for Research on Cancer

IDLH: immediately dangerous to life or health

JCAHO: Joint Commission on Accreditation of Healthcare Organizations

LEPC: local emergency planning committee

LSC: *Life Safety Code®*

LSO: laser safety officer

MPE: maximum permissible exposure

MSD: musculoskeletal disorder

MSDS: material safety data sheets

NFPA: National Fire Protection Association

NHZ: nominal hazard zone

NIOSH: National Institute for Occupational Safety and Health

NM: nanometer

NRC: Nuclear Regulatory Commission

NTP: National Toxicology Program

OPIM: other potentially infectious material

OSHA: Occupational Safety and Health Administration

PACM: presumed asbestos-containing materials

PAPR: powered air-purifying respirator

PEL: permissible exposure limit

PPE: personal protective equipment

PPM: parts per million

PSI: pounds per square inch

QLFT: qualitative fit test

QNFT: quantitative fit test

RCRA: Resource Conservation and Recovery Act

SARA: Superfund Amendments Reauthorization Act

SCBA: self-contained breathing apparatus

SOP: standard operating procedure

STEL: short-term exposure limit

STS: standard threshold shift

TB: tuberculosis

TLV: threshold limit value

TSD: treatment, storage, and disposal (facility)

TSI: thermal systems insulation

TWA: time-weighted average

UP: universal precautions

Access to records (1904, 1910, 1020, 1913.10, and others)

at a glance

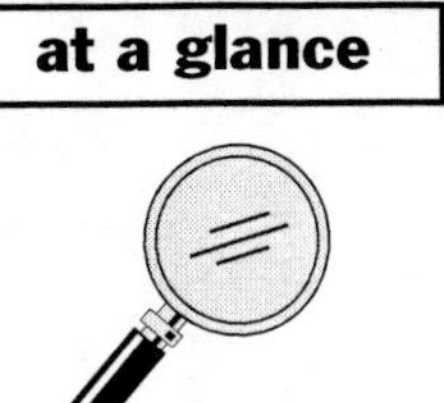

Records must be made available upon request to current or former employees, employee representatives, OSHA, and NIOSH for examination and copying. Records must be preserved and maintained. Confidentiality issues are addressed.

Under 29 CFR 1910.1020, requirements apply to the maintenance and retention of records for medical surveillance, exposure monitoring, inspections, and other activities and incidents relevant to occupational safety and health.

Individual health records must be kept in the employee health-service department. OSHA defines an employee medical record as one that concerns the health status of an employee and is made or maintained by a physician, registered nurse, or other healthcare professional or technician. Each employee health record must be maintained for the duration of employment plus 30 years, unless a specific occupational safety and health standard requires a different period of time. Laboratory reports and worksheets need to be kept for only one year.

Employers are required to maintain accurate records of certain potentially toxic or harmful physical agents that must be monitored or measured. Employers must promptly advise employees of any excessive exposure and the corrective action taken. In certain cases, physical examinations and testing are required. OSHA requires that the employee exposure records be maintained for the duration of employment plus 30 years. Employees or their designated representatives have a right to review their individual employee medical records and records that describe employee exposures.

When employees request their exposure records, the employer is required to furnish them within 15 days. Employee representatives also may examine and copy a worker's exposure records. If prescribed procedures are followed, OSHA has the right to see exposure records.

Confidentiality

Employee health records must be treated with the level of confidentiality necessary to protect employee privacy. The employer must make the records available to the employee—or authorized representative—if requested by the employee. Employees or their representatives have the right to examine and copy the results of exposure monitoring.

The employee exposure record must also contain the following:

- Environmental monitoring, specific sampling results, the collection methodology, a description of the analytical and mathematical methods used, and a summary of other background data relevant to interpretation of the results obtained

- Biological monitoring results that directly assess the absorption of a hazard

- MSDSs or a hazard inventory that describes chemicals and identifies where and when they are used

Exemptions

The following types of records are exempt from the retention rule:

- Health-insurance claims maintained separately from the employer's medical program and its records

- First-aid records of one-time treatment and subsequent observation

- Medical records of employees who have worked for less than one year for the employer need not be retained beyond the term of employment if they are provided to the employee upon termination

- Records that concern voluntary EAPs (alcohol, drug abuse, or personal counseling), if maintained separately from the employer's medical program and its records

Additional requirements

The records-access standard also includes the following provisions:

- The storage of information in any form—document, microfilm, x-ray, or automated data processing—is permitted, but chest x-rays must be kept in their original state

- Employer trade secrets should conform with OSHA's hazard-communication standard

- Employee representatives (such as union representatives) must show an occupational health need for requested records when seeking access to employee exposure records without consent

Similar provisions apply to employees' medical records. However, for privacy interests, employee representatives are allowed access to the records only with written consent of the employee concerned. The records-access rule requires that employees be informed upon employment, and annually thereafter, of their rights of access to the records and the correct procedures for exercising those rights.

Air contaminants (1910.1000)

at a glance

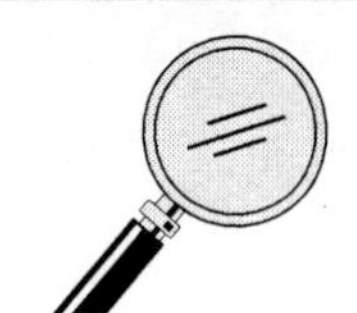

The air contaminants standard sets exposure limits for hundreds of substances contained in gases, fumes, and dust, and requires monitoring.

Air contaminants

Laboratory employees may be exposed at times to a variety of harmful materials in the air, including gases, dusts, mists, vapors, fumes, and other substances.

OSHA issued the air-contaminants standard to require employers to monitor employee exposure to potentially harmful chemicals and other airborne substances, and to keep such exposures within permissible limits. Employers that fail to comply with the air-contaminants standard could be subject to enforcement action.

Employers also are required to provide hazard information and training to employees who may be exposed to chemicals covered under the air-contaminants standard.

Regulated substances

Chemical substances used in healthcare facilities and regulated under the air-contaminants standard include

- mercury
- methyl methacrylate
- methanol
- xylene
- ammonia
- chlorine
- chlorofluorocarbons or Freon™

To comply with the air-contaminants standard, employers should take an inventory of each work-site to determine whether hazardous air contaminants are present, the levels of such contaminants, and how they can be controlled or mitigated as required.

Permissible exposure limits (PEL)

The air-contaminants standard specifies PELs for hundreds of potentially hazardous chemicals and other substances. PELs are based on three different increments of time:

- An eight-hour measurement taken to determine the TWA
- A 15-minute measurement for a STEL
- An instantaneous measurement for the ceiling limit

Many PELs have not been updated in years and are considered by some safety experts to be too permissive to adequately protect workers. Some experts advise employers to reduce the likelihood of endangering workers and being cited for a safety violation by using exposure limits adopted by OSHA for the purpose of updating the standard in 1989. Alternatively, employers may wish to follow current recommendations of the ACGIH or NIOSH.

Monitoring methods

Tools commonly used to obtain required measurements include

- personal dosimeters/monitoring badges
- detector tubes
- industrial hygiene methods, such as vacuum pumps and a variety of filter media

More sophisticated means include use of portable gas chromatographs and infrared spectrophotometers.

Recordkeeping requirements

All air-monitoring data must be recorded and retained by the employer for a minimum of 30 years. These records also must be made available to employees in accordance with OSHA requirements.

Required exposure controls

Employers are required to enable administrative or engineering controls to bring employee exposure levels within permissible limits. Only in cases where such controls are not feasible may PPE and other measures be used to meet the PELs.

All control measures must be approved for that specific use by a competent industrial hygienist or other technically qualified person.

Hierarchy of controls

Industrial hygienists commonly follow a system known as the "hierarchy of controls" to ensure that the most consistent means of controlling a hazard is used wherever possible. The system ranks controls in descending order of consistency and overall effectiveness. An example of this approach would be installation of local-exhaust ventilation to remove glutaraldehyde fumes from a medical sterilization area, rather than simply requiring employees to wear respirators when working there.

The air-contaminants standard requires employers to institute the hierarchy of controls to a certain extent, as engineering and administrative controls must be used wherever possible before work-practice and other controls may be relied upon to meet the PELs. However, the regulation in some cases allows employers to rely upon employee rotation—an administrative control—to limit exposures to hazardous substances. This method is rejected by many safety experts as inconsistent with the goal of reducing hazardous exposures for the greatest number of employees.

Control methods

Employee exposure to air contaminants can be prevented or reduced through various control methods:

- Elimination of the hazard (e.g., by contracting with an outside firm that provides services such as medical-instrument sterilization).

- Substitution of less-toxic materials.

- Change of a process.
  - Isolation (e.g., placing the hazardous process in a separate room or in a corner of the building to reduce the number of persons exposed).
  - Engineering controls are used to control a hazard at the source. Primary examples include local-exhaust ventilation, general dilution ventilation, and closed systems.

- Administrative controls (e.g., limiting the total amount of time an individual is exposed to a health hazard, or rotating two or more workers each day).

- Training and information—Employees should be told what hazards they are exposed to and the safe-work practices they should use to reduce or limit exposure.

- Personal hygiene—Employees who are exposed to hazardous substances should wash their hands before eating, smoking, or using toilet facilities. Skin exposed to chemicals such as alkalies, acids, solvents, and strong cleaning agents should be washed immediately. Employees should not be permitted to eat around toxic chemicals or in contaminated areas. Clothing should be changed and washed daily if it becomes contaminated with toxic chemicals, dusts, fumes, or liquids.

- PPE—Items such as respirators, protective clothing, and protective equipment must be made available. The items should be provided and maintained in compliance with OSHA requirements for PPE.

Identifying hazardous substances

Often, health hazards associated with air contaminants are not recognized because materials used in them are identified only by trade names. A further complication arises from the fact that materials tend to contain mixtures of substances, which makes identification difficult. To identify occupational health hazards in a particular workplace, a materials analysis should be conducted at each operation to show all chemicals used and all products and byproducts formed. All hazardous substances should then be listed and evaluated. The most likely mode of exposure should be noted (e.g., ingestion, skin absorption, or inhalation). Most of this information is available on the MSDS that is supplied with the product upon purchase or delivery.

After this analysis is completed, related activities such as maintenance and service operations should be examined for health-hazard potential. Control measures should be activated where necessary to keep exposure within permissible or recommended limits.

Asbestos (1910.1001 for general industry and 1926.1101 for construction)

at a glance

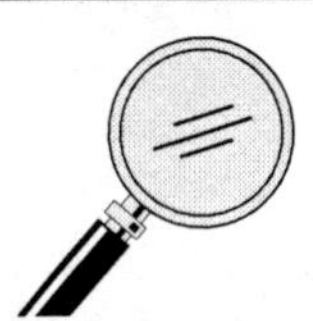

The asbestos standard protects workers from asbestos exposure.

Asbestos includes chrysotile, amosite, crocidolite, tremolite asbestos, anthophyllite asbestos, actinolite asbestos, and chemically treated or altered versions of these minerals. The definition under general industry and construction standards does not include nonasbestiform varieties of the minerals tremolite, anthophyllite, and actinolite.

Standards for protecting workers from exposure to asbestos in construction, general industry, and shipyard employment were revised and reissued by OSHA in August 1994. The PELs for airborne asbestos are 0.1 fiber per cubic centimeter (f/cc) of air as an eight-hour TWA and 1.0 f/cc averaged over 30 minutes as a STEL.

Laboratory employers may be affected by construction activities and/or general industry rules. Both have provisions for exposure monitoring, respiratory protection, employee training, and recordkeeping. But the standards have major differences as well.

The construction-activities standard (29 CFR 1926.1101) covers asbestos hazards related to demolition, renovation, or maintenance, regardless of the employer's primary business. Such work is divided into classes (Class I, II, III, and IV) that correspond to the levels of exposure hazard. The extent of controls required depends upon the classification of the work.

Generally, however, employers must

- appoint a competent person to supervise asbestos-related work
- conduct initial exposure monitoring at the start of each asbestos job
- establish regulated areas for asbestos jobs, with posted warnings and restricted access

- use wet methods to control fiber dispersion during asbestos work and HEPA high-efficiency particulate air-filter vacuums to clean up asbestos dust and debris

- ensure prompt disposal of asbestos-containing material

The general industry standard (29 CFR 1910.1001) covers most nonconstruction exposure. Employers generally are required to

- provide housekeeping and other employees with information and training on the location of asbestos hazards in the facility

- conduct initial monitoring for employees who are or may be exposed above the PELs

- institute a written plan for reducing exposure through engineering and other controls where exposure exceeds the PELs

General-industry asbestos standard

Scope of coverage

The OSHA asbestos standard for general industry (29 CFR 1910.1001) applies to all activities, except agriculture, that are not otherwise covered by the construction-asbestos or shipyard-employment standards.

PELs

OSHA sets the PEL for airborne asbestos at 0.1 f/cc of air as an eight-hour TWA. For short-term exposure, the excursion limit is 1 f/cc as averaged over a 30-minute sampling period.

Monitoring requirements

The asbestos standard for general industry contains provisions for initial and periodic exposure monitoring.

Initial monitoring

Employers are required to conduct initial exposure monitoring for employees who are or may reasonably be expected to be exposed above the TWA PEL or the excursion limit. In cases where the employer conducted monitoring after March 31, 1992, for the TWA or the excursion limit, and the monitoring met the standard's requirements, the employer may rely on these earlier results to satisfy the initial monitoring requirement. No initial monitoring is required where the employer has relied on objective data that show that asbestos cannot be released at or above the TWA PEL under expected conditions of use or handling.

Periodic monitoring

Samples must be taken at least every six months for employees whose exposures may exceed the TWA PEL or excursion limit. If either the initial or periodic monitoring shows that employee exposures are below the TWA PEL or the excursion limit, the employer may discontinue monitoring for those employees.

Additional monitoring is required whenever there is a change in production or processes that could result in new or additional exposures above the TWA PEL or excursion limit or if the employer has any reason to suspect that a change may result in new or additional exposures above the PEL or the excursion limit.

Determinations of employee exposure should be made by taking breathing-zone air samples that are representative of the eight-hour TWA and 30-minute short-term exposures of each employee. Representative eight-hour TWA employee exposures must be based on one or more samples that represent the exposure for each employee working a full shift. Representative 30-minute short-term exposures must be based on one or more samples of 30-minute exposures associated with work that is most likely to produce exposures above the excursion limit.

Monitoring methods

All samples taken to satisfy the monitoring requirements must be personal samples collected following procedures specified in Appendix A of the standard. All samples taken must be evaluated using the OSHA Reference Method or an equivalent counting method that satisfies OSHA requirements.

Employee notification

The employer must notify employees of the monitoring results in writing or by posting in an appropriate place within 15 days after receipt of the results. The written notification must contain the corrective action being taken by the employer to reduce employee exposure to or below the TWA and/or the excursion limit wherever monitoring results indicated that the TWA and/or excursion limit had been exceeded. Employees are permitted to observe monitoring but must use proper protective equipment.

Regulated areas

The employer is required to establish regulated areas wherever airborne concentrations of asbestos are in excess of the TWA and/or excursion limit. These areas should be marked off from the rest of the workplace in a way that minimizes the number of persons who will be exposed. Access to regulated areas must be limited to authorized persons.

Each person who enters a regulated area must be supplied with and required to use an appropriate respirator. The employer must make sure employees do not eat, drink, smoke, chew tobacco or gum, or apply cosmetics in these regulated areas.

Methods of compliance

Employers are required to institute engineering controls and work practices to reduce and maintain employee exposure at or below the TWA and/or excursion limit to the extent feasible. Whenever feasible engineering controls and work practices are not enough to reduce exposure to permissible levels, appropriate respiratory protection must be used. Local-exhaust ventilation and dust-collection systems must be designed, constructed, installed, and maintained in accordance with American National Standard Fundamentals Governing the Design and Operation of Local Exhaust Systems (ANSI Z 9.2-1979). All hand- and power-operated tools—such as saws, scorers, and drills—that would produce or release asbestos fibers should be provided with local-exhaust ventilation systems that meet the ANSI standards.

Where practical, asbestos must be handled, mixed, applied, removed, cut, scored, or otherwise worked in a wet state sufficient to prevent the emission of airborne fibers.

Products such as cement, mortar, grout, plaster, and similar materials that contain asbestos should not be removed from shipping containers without being wetted, ventilated, or enclosed so as to prevent the release of airborne fibers.

Compressed air may not be used to remove asbestos unless it is used in conjunction with a ventilation system designed to capture the dust cloud created by the compressed air.

Written compliance program

Where the TWA or excursion limit is exceeded, the employer must establish a written program to reduce employee exposure to permissible levels through the use of engineering and work-practice controls and respirators where appropriate.

The program must be reviewed and updated regularly and be available upon request to OSHA, affected employees, and their representatives.

Job rotation may not be used as a means of complying with the TWA and excursion limits.

Respiratory protection

OSHA's general-industry standard for asbestos includes respiratory-protection provisions (29 CFR 1910.1001[g]) for employees who use respirators for asbestos-related activities.

Employers must provide the respirators and ensure that they are used during

- periods necessary to install feasible engineering and work-practice controls
- work operations, such as maintenance and repair activities, for which engineering and work-practice controls are not feasible
- work operations for which feasible engineering and work-practice controls are not yet sufficient to reduce exposure at or below the TWA and/or excursion limit

Respirator program

Where respiratory protection is required, the employer must create a respirator program in accordance with applicable requirements of OSHA's respiratory protection standard at 29 CFR 1910.134.

No employee may be assigned to tasks that require the use of respirators if, based on the most recent medical examination, the examining physician determines that the employee will be unable to function normally using a respirator. In this case, the employee must be assigned to another job or given the opportunity to transfer to a different job. If a transfer is available, the position must be with the same employer; in the same geographical area; and with the same seniority, status, and rate of pay the employee had immediately prior to the transfer.

Respirator selection

When certain airborne concentrations of asbestos or conditions of use are encountered in the work environment, the employer must select and provide the appropriate respirator as specified in Table 1 at the end of this chapter.

The employer must provide a tight-fitting PAPR instead of any negative-pressure respirator when an employee chooses to use this type of respirator, as long as the PAPR provides adequate protection.

Respirator fit testing

Under the respiratory-protection standard (29 CFR 1910.134[f]), before an employee may be required to use any respirator with a negative- or positive-pressure tight-fitting facepiece, the employee must be fit tested with the same make, model, style, and size of respirator to be used. Such employees must pass an appropriate qualitative or quantitative fit test prior to initial use of the respirator, whenever a different respirator facepiece is used, and at least annually thereafter. Additional fit tests may be required as necessary.

Additional requirements

The respiratory-protection standard also includes requirements for respirator use, maintenance, and care; breathing air quality and use; identification of filters, cartridges, and canisters; employee training and information; respirator program evaluation; employee medical evaluation; and recordkeeping.

Protective clothing and equipment

If an employee is exposed to asbestos above the TWA and/or the excursion limit, or where the possibility of eye irritation exists, the employer must provide, at no cost to the employee, protective work clothing and equipment. Examples of such items include the following:

- Coveralls or similar full-body work clothing
- Gloves, head coverings, and foot coverings
- Face shields, vented goggles, or other appropriate protective equipment

Contaminated clothing must not be taken out of the change room, except by employees authorized to do so for the purpose of laundering, maintenance, or disposal. Contaminated work clothing must be placed and stored in closed containers to prevent the dispersion of asbestos. These containers must be labeled appropriately. Employers may not allow employees to remove asbestos from protective clothing or equipment by shaking or blowing. Employers must clean, launder, repair, or replace protective clothing and equipment for, and provide clean protective clothing and equipment to, each affected employee at least weekly.

Laundering contaminated clothing must be done in a manner that does not release airborne fibers above the PELs, and those performing the service must be informed of this requirement.

Hygiene facilities

OSHA regulations require that hygiene facilities be made available to workers who may be exposed to asbestos. Required facilities include

- change rooms with separate lockers for street clothes and asbestos-contaminated clothing.
- showers for employees who work in areas where the TWA and/or the excursion limit is exceeded. Showers must be taken at the end of each work shift.
- lunchrooms for employees who work in areas where PELs are exceeded. Employees must wash their hands and faces prior to eating, drinking, or smoking.

Employees may not be allowed to enter the lunch room with protective work clothing or equipment unless surface fibers have been removed by vacuuming or another method that removes dust without causing asbestos fibers to become airborne.

Communication of hazards: Disclosure of asbestos-containing materials

Exposure to asbestos in general industry can occur in a variety of settings, including housekeeping activities in public or commercial buildings that contain installed ACM (e.g., flooring).

Housekeeping employees should know whether the building components they maintain will expose them to asbestos, according to OSHA.

Because building owners are often the best and/or only source of information concerning the presence of previously installed ACM, the asbestos standard assigns to them and to employers of potentially exposed workers responsibilities for conveying hazard information. Specifically, the standard requires building and facility owners to

- determine the presence, location, and quantity of ACM and PACM at the work site
- inform employers of the presence and location of ACM and/or PACM in areas where they may be contacted during housekeeping activities, so employers may inform employees who perform such activities in those areas
- maintain records of all information required or known that concern the presence, location, and quantity of ACM and PACM

PACM

Installed thermal system insulation and sprayed-on and troweled-on surfacing materials in buildings constructed in 1980 or earlier must be treated as PACM. Asphalt and vinyl flooring material installed in 1980 or earlier must also be treated as asbestos-containing, unless the employer or building owner demonstrates otherwise in accordance with the standard.

Demonstrate that PACM does not contain asbestos by completing an inspection in accordance with the EPA's Asbestos Hazard Emergency Response Act regulations (40 CFR 763, Subpart E); performing tests on bulk samples by an accredited inspector or certified industrial hygienist; or, in the case of flooring material, receiving determination by an industrial hygienist based on recognized analytical techniques.

Due diligence

Employers and building and facility owners must exercise due diligence in complying with the requirements to inform employers and employees about the presence and location of ACM and PACM. The term "due diligence" is not defined in the asbestos standard, but OSHA states that a reasonable employer, informed of the asbestos standard and other pertinent regulations, must inquire into the possibility that a building material is asbestos-containing. The required extent of the inquiry may vary, depending on the prevalence of ACM in that location, previous surveys, inspections, other knowledge sources, and the date the material was installed, OSHA says.

Warning signs and labels

Warning signs must be provided and displayed at each regulated area. They also must be posted at all approaches to regulated areas so that employees can protect themselves before entering the area.

The warning signs must state the following:

DANGER
ASBESTOS
CANCER AND LUNG DISEASE HAZARD
AUTHORIZED PERSONNEL ONLY

In addition, where the use of respirators and protective clothing is required in the regulated area, the warning signs must state the following:

RESPIRATORS
AND PROTECTIVE CLOTHING
ARE REQUIRED IN THIS AREA

Employers must ensure that employees who work in or around regulated areas understand the warning signs. Means to ensure employee comprehension may include the use of foreign languages, pictographs, and graphics.

At the entrance to mechanical rooms/areas that employees enter and that contain ACM/PACM, the building owner must post signs that identify the material present, its location, and work practices that will ensure that the ACM or PACM is not disturbed. Employers must ensure that employees can comprehend the signs. Comprehension may necessitate the use of foreign languages, pictographs, graphics, and awareness training.

Warning labels must be put on all products that contain asbestos fibers, as well as their containers.

Labels must comply with the requirements of OSHA's hazard communication standard (29 CFR 1910.1200[f]) and include the following information:

DANGER
CONTAINS ASBESTOS FIBERS
AVOID CREATING DUST
CANCER AND LUNG DISEASE HAZARD

When a building owner or employer identifies previously installed ACM and/or PACM, labels or signs must be posted where they will clearly be noticed by employees likely to be exposed (e.g., at the entrance to mechanical room/areas). This will satisfy OSHA's requirement as long as the signs contain information required for labels. Employers must make sure that employees can comprehend the signs. Comprehension may necessitate the use of foreign languages, pictographs, graphics, and awareness training.

Housekeeping

OSHA requires employers to comply with specific housekeeping provisions that include the following:

- All surfaces must be maintained as free of ACM waste and debris and accompanying dust as possible
- Spills and sudden releases of material that contain asbestos must be cleaned up as soon as possible
- Surfaces contaminated by asbestos may not be cleaned using compressed air
- HEPA-filtered vacuuming equipment should be used to vacuum asbestos-containing waste and debris
- Shoveling, dry sweeping, and dry cleanup of asbestos may be used only where vacuuming and/or wet cleaning are not feasible

Asbestos-containing flooring material should be cared for only in accordance with the following provisions:

- Sanding of asbestos-containing flooring material is prohibited
- Stripping of finishes should be conducted using low-abrasion pads at speeds lower than 300 revolutions per minute and using wet methods
- Burnishing or dry buffing may be performed only on asbestos-containing flooring that contains sufficient finish to prevent the pad from contacting the ACM
- Waste and debris and accompanying dust in an area that contains accessible ACM and/or PACM or visibly deteriorated ACM may not be dusted, swept dry, or vacuumed without using a HEPA filter

Medical surveillance

Employers must institute a medical-surveillance program for all employees who are, or will be, exposed to airborne concentrations of asbestos fibers at or above the action level and/or the excursion limit. Medical examinations must be performed under the supervision of a licensed physician, and must be provided without cost to the employee. Pulmonary-function testing must be performed by a person trained in spirometry. Preplacement examinations are required before an employee is assigned to an occupation that exposes him or her to airborne asbestos fibers. This examination must include, at a minimum, a medical and work history; a complete physical exam of all systems, with emphasis on the respiratory system, the cardiovascular system, and digestive tract; completion of the respiratory-disease standardized questionnaire; a chest roentgenogram; a pulmonary-function test; and any other tests deemed appropriate.

Periodic examinations must be made available annually. The frequency of chest roentgenograms must be conducted according to Table 2 at the end of this chapter.

Termination-of-employment examinations must be provided for any employee who has been exposed to airborne concentrations of asbestos fibers at or above the action level and/or the excursion limit.

The medical examination must be in accordance with the requirements of the periodic examination and must be given 30 calendar days before or after the date of termination of employment.

No medical examination is required of any employees whose records show that they have been appropriately examined within the past one-year period.

The employer must obtain a written, signed opinion from the examining physician that contains the results of the medical examination and must provide the affected employee with a copy of the opinion within 30 days of its receipt.

The employer must establish and maintain an accurate record for each employee subject to medical surveillance and maintain it for the duration of employment plus 30 years, except for short-term employees.

Training

The general-industry asbestos standard details training requirements for employees. Employees who will be exposed at or above the PELs must be provided training prior to or at the time of initial assignment and at least annually thereafter. Training must be conducted in a manner that employees understand and must encompass the following:

- The health effects associated with asbestos exposure
- Increased risk of cancer when one combines smoking and exposure to asbestos
- The amount, location, manner of use, release, and storage of asbestos, and the kinds of operations that can result in asbestos exposure

- Engineering controls and work practices associated with the employee's job
- Specific procedures used to protect employees from exposure (e.g., work practices, emergency and cleanup procedures, and PPE to be used)
- The purpose, use, and limitations of respirators and protective clothing
- The purpose and description of the medical surveillance program required by the standard
- The contents of OSHA's asbestos standard, including appendices
- The names and telephone numbers of public health organizations that offer smoking cessation programs (e.g., the list contained in Appendix I of the standard)
- The sign-posting and labeling requirements of the standard and the meaning of required legends for signs and labels

Employees who perform housekeeping in an area that has ACM or PACM must be provided free-of-charge asbestos-awareness training. The course must be provided annually and must contain the following elements:

- Health effects of asbestos
- Locations of ACM and PACM in the facility
- Recognition of ACM/PACM damage and deterioration
- The standard's requirements related to housekeeping
- Proper response to fiber-release episodes

The employer must keep all employee training records for one year beyond the last date of employment of each employee.

Construction asbestos standard

Scope of coverage

Coverage under the construction-activities asbestos standard (29 CFR 1926.1101) is based on the nature of the work that involves asbestos exposure, not on the primary activity of the employer. Generally, the standard applies to maintenance and other workers involved in activities that include

- demolition or salvage of structures where asbestos is present
- removal or encapsulation of materials that contain asbestos
- construction, alteration, repair, maintenance, or renovation of structures, substrates, or portions thereof that contain asbestos
- installation of products that contain asbestos
- spill or emergency cleanup of asbestos
- transportation, disposal, storage, containment of, and housekeeping activities that involve asbestos or products that contain asbestos on the site or location at which construction activities are performed

Certain provisions also apply to workers at multi-employer work sites who may be exposed to asbestos due to their proximity to asbestos construction activities. PELs under the construction standard are the same as for general industry: a TWA of 0.1 f/cc and an excursion limit 1 f/cc.

Work classifications

The construction standard has taken a new approach in protecting workers exposed to asbestos. Rather than relying on measured exposure levels to determine coverage, the standard's provisions are triggered by the type of work being done. Such work is divided into four classes of construction activities based on varying hazard levels and matched, in descending order, with appropriate control requirements. These classifications are defined as follows:

- **Class I**: Removal of TSI and surfacing (i.e., sprayed-on or troweled-on ACM and PACM).
- **Class II**: Removal of ACM or PACM that is not TSI or surfacing ACM or PACM.
- **Class III**: Repair and maintenance operations that are likely to disturb ACM or PACM. This includes maintenance work where a small amount of ACM must be cut away to access a building's structural or mechanical components, according to OSHA. A "small amount" is a quantity that can be contained in a standard-sized glove bag or waste bag if the bag is 1/3 to 1/2 full, as it should be to allow secure closure and reduce risk of breakage.
- **Class IV**: Maintenance, custodial, and housekeeping activities during which employees contact but do not disturb ACM or PACM and activities to clean up dust, waste, and debris that results from Class I, II, and III activities.

Regulated areas

All Class I, II, and III asbestos work must be done in regulated areas. Other operations must be done in regulated areas when airborne concentrations of asbestos exceed or may exceed PELs. All asbestos work performed in regulated areas must be supervised by what OSHA terms a "competent person." The regulated area must be marked off in a way that minimizes the number of people within the area and protects individuals outside the area from exposure to airborne asbestos. Access to regulated areas must be limited to authorized persons.

Designation of a competent person

Employers must ensure that all asbestos work performed in regulated areas is supervised by a competent person. This person should have the qualifications and authority necessary to ensure worker safety as required in OSHA's General Safety and Health Provisions for Construction

(29 CFR 1926.20–1926.32). The competent person's duties include frequent and regular inspections of job sites, materials, and equipment. For Class I and II asbestos work, additional duties include setting up regulated areas, ensuring the integrity of enclosures and containments, supervising employee-exposure monitoring, and ensuring that safe work practices are followed and PPE is used as required.

A competent person is defined in the standard as one who is capable of identifying existing asbestos hazards in the workplace and selecting the appropriate control strategy for asbestos exposure, and who has the authority to eliminate them. For Class I and Class II work, a competent person is one who is specially trained in a course that meets the EPA's Model Accreditation Plan or its equivalent; for Class III and Class IV work, it is one who is trained in a manner consistent with EPA requirements for training of local education agency maintenance and custodial staff under 40 CFR 763.92(a)(2). Additional OSHA training requirements for the competent person are found at 29 CFR 1926.1101(o)(4).

Multi-employer work sites

The responsibilities of contractors and other employers involved in activities at the same work site are detailed in the construction asbestos standard.

Generally, the contractor who creates or controls the asbestos hazard is responsible for abating the hazard. Additionally, employers must take steps to protect their employees who are exposed to the hazard. More specifically, the standard states that on multi-employer work sites,

- the employer who performs work in a regulated area must inform other employers on the site of the nature of the work with asbestos, the existence of and requirements relating to regulated areas, and the measures taken to ensure that employees of other employers are not exposed to asbestos.

- the contractor who created or controls the source of asbestos contamination is responsible for abating the asbestos hazards.

- all employers of exposed employees must comply with applicable protective provisions for their employees. For example, if employees who work immediately adjacent to a Class I asbestos job are exposed to asbestos due to the inadequate containment of the job, their employer is required either to remove the employees from the area or to perform initial exposure assessment as required under the standard.

- all employers of employees who work adjacent to regulated areas established by another employer on a multi-employer work site are required to take steps daily to ascertain the integrity of the enclosure and/or the effectiveness of the contractor's primary control method for ensuring that asbestos fibers do not migrate to adjacent areas.

- all general contractors on a construction project exercise general supervisory authority over the work covered by the standard. The general contractor is required to ascertain whether the asbestos contractor is in compliance with the construction asbestos standard and must require the contractor to come into compliance with the standard when necessary.

Exposure assessment and monitoring

The asbestos standard for construction activities contains provisions for initial and periodic exposure monitoring.

Initial monitoring

All employers that have a workplace covered by this standard must conduct an initial exposure assessment at the beginning of each asbestos job to predict whether exposure levels will exceed the PELs and whether more monitoring and other precautions will be needed.

The employer must make sure that a competent person conducts the initial exposure assessment immediately before or at the start of the work to determine what level of asbestos exposure to expect.

Determination of employee exposure must be made from breathing-zone air samples that are representative of the eight-hour TWA and 30-minute short-term exposures of each employee.

For any specific job that will be performed by employees who have been trained in compliance with the standard, the employer may show that employees will be exposed below the PEL, resulting in a negative-exposure assessment.

Periodic monitoring

For Class I and II operations, the employer must conduct daily monitoring, unless the employer has made a negative-exposure assessment. For Class III and IV operations, the employer must conduct periodic monitoring of all work where exposures are expected to exceed the PEL.

If periodic monitoring shows that employee exposures are below the PELs, the employer may discontinue monitoring for those employees. However, the employer must institute exposure monitoring any time there has been a change in process, control equipment, personnel, or work practices that may result in new or additional exposure above the TWA or excursion limit, or when the employer has any reason to suspect that a change may result in new or additional exposures. This additional monitoring is required whether or not a negative-exposure assessment was previously produced.

Methods of compliance

The employer must use the following engineering controls and work practices, regardless of the levels of exposure:

- Vacuum cleaners equipped with HEPA filters to collect all debris and dust that contains ACM or PACM

- Wet methods, or wetting agents, to control employee exposures during asbestos handling, except where employers show that the use of wet methods is infeasible (e.g., due to the creation of electrical hazards, equipment malfunctions, and slipping hazards)

- Prompt cleanup and disposal of wastes and debris contaminated with asbestos in leak-tight containers

The employer also must use the following control methods to comply with the TWA PEL and excursion limit:

- Local-exhaust ventilation equipped with HEPA filter dust-collection systems
- Enclosure or isolation of processes that produce asbestos dust
- Ventilation of the regulated area to move contaminated air away from the breathing zone and toward a filtration device equipped with a HEPA filter

High-speed abrasive disc saws, compressed air, dry sweeping, and employee rotation as a means of reducing asbestos exposure cannot be used for asbestos work.

Classes I, II, III, and IV each have additional engineering controls and work practices detailed in the standard.

Additional exemptions and requirements that apply to removal of asbestos-containing roofing materials are detailed in the standard.

Respiratory protection

OSHA's construction-industry standard for asbestos includes respiratory protection provisions (29 CFR 1926.1101[h]) for employees who use respirators for asbestos-related activities. The employer must provide the respirators and ensure that they are used during the following:

- Class I asbestos work
- Class II asbestos work when ACM is not removed in a substantially intact state

- Class II and III asbestos work that is not performed using wet methods (except during removal of ACM from sloped roofs if a negative-exposure assessment results and the ACM is removed in an intact state)
- Class II and III asbestos work for which a negative-exposure assessment has not been conducted
- Class III work when TSI or surfacing ACM or PACM is being disturbed
- Class IV work performed within regulated areas where employees who perform other work are required to wear respirators
- Work operations for which employees are exposed above the TWA or excursion limit
- Emergencies

Respirator program

Where respiratory protection is required, the employer must create a respirator program in accordance with applicable requirements of OSHA's respiratory protection standard at 29 CFR 1910.134.

No employee may be assigned to tasks requiring the use of respirators if, based on the most recent medical examination, the examining physician determines that the employee will be unable to function normally using a respirator. In this case, the employee must be assigned to another job or given the opportunity to transfer to a job that he or she can perform. If such a transfer is available, the position must be with the same employer, in the same geographical area, and with the same seniority, status, and rate of pay the employee had immediately prior to the transfer.

Respirator selection

When certain airborne concentrations of asbestos or conditions of use are encountered in the work environment, the employer must select and provide the appropriate respirator as specified in Table 3 at the end of this chapter.

Whenever an employee chooses to use a tight-fitting PAPR in place of a negative-pressure respirator, the employer must provide the PAPR, as long as it provides adequate protection.

Employers are required to provide a half-mask air-purifying respirator (not a disposable respirator) equipped with high-efficiency filters whenever an employee performs Class II and III asbestos work when a negative-exposure assessment has not been conducted or Class III jobs when thermal systems insulation or surfacing ACM or PACM is disturbed.

In addition, when employees are in a regulated area where Class I work is being performed, a negative-exposure assessment of the area has not been produced, and the exposure assessment of the area indicates the exposure level will not exceed 1 f/cc as an eight-hour TWA, employers must provide the employees with one of the following respirators:

- A tight-fitting PAPR equipped with high-efficiency filters.
- A full-facepiece supplied-air respirator operated in the pressure-demand mode equipped with HEPA egress cartridges.
- A full-facepiece supplied-air respirator operated in the pressure-demand mode equipped with an auxiliary positive-pressure self-contained breathing apparatus (SCBA). This type of respirator must be provided when the exposure assessment indicates exposure levels above 1 f/cc as an eight-hour TWA.

Respirator fit testing

Under the respiratory-protection standard (29 CFR 1910.134[f]), before an employee may be required to use any respirator with a negative- or positive-pressure tight-fitting facepiece, the employee must be fit tested with the same make, model, style, and size of respirator to be used. Such employees must pass an appropriate qualitative or quantitative fit test prior to initial use of the respirator, whenever a different respirator facepiece is used, and at least annually thereafter. Additional fit tests may be required as necessary.

Additional requirements

The respiratory-protection standard also includes requirements for respirator use, maintenance, and care; breathing air quality and use; identification of filters, cartridges, and canisters; employee training and information; respirator-program evaluation; employee medical evaluation; and recordkeeping.

Hygiene facilities and practices

For employees who perform Class I asbestos jobs that involve more than 25 linear or 10 square feet of TSI or surfacing ACM and PACM, the employer must establish a decontamination area that is adjacent and connected to the regulated area. The decontamination area must consist of an equipment room, shower area, and clean room. The employer must ensure that employees enter and exit the regulated area through the decontamination area.

The clean room must be equipped with a locker or appropriate storage area for each employee. The shower area should be contiguous both to the equipment room and the clean change room, but if this is not possible, the employer must make sure that employees remove contamination from their worksuits using a HEPA vacuum before proceeding to the shower. The equipment room must be supplied with impermeable, labeled bags and containers for containment and disposal of contaminated clothing and protective equipment.

Decontamination area entry procedures

The employer must ensure that employees

- enter the decontamination area through the clean room
- remove and deposit street clothing in the storage provided
- put on protective clothing and respiratory protection before leaving the clean room
- pass through the equipment room before entering the regulated area

Decontamination area exit procedures

The employer must ensure that, before leaving the regulated area, employees

- remove all gross contamination and debris from protective clothing
- remove their protective clothing in the equipment room and deposit the clothing in labeled, impermeable bags or containers
- do not remove their respirators in the equipment room
- shower prior to entering the clean room
- enter the clean room before changing to street clothes

For Class I work that involves less than 25 linear or 10 square feet of TSI or surfacing ACM and PACM, and for Class II and Class III operations where exposures exceed PELs, employers must establish an equipment room that consists of an area covered by an impermeable drop cloth. Work clothing must be cleaned with a HEPA vacuum before it is removed, and all equipment and surfaces of containers filled with ACM must be cleaned before they are removed from the equipment room. The employer must ensure that employees enter and exit the regulated area through the equipment room.

For Class IV work, employers must ensure that employees comply with the hygiene practice required of employees who perform work with a higher classification within that regulated area.

Communication of hazards

Warning signs that mark the regulated areas must be provided at each location. Signs must be posted at a distance that allows employees to read the signs and take necessary protective steps before entering the area.

The warning signs for regulated areas must contain the following information:

DANGER
ASBESTOS
CANCER AND LUNG DISEASE HAZARD
AUTHORIZED PERSONNEL ONLY

In addition, where the use of respirators and protective clothing is required, the warning signs must state the following:

RESPIRATORS AND PROTECTIVE CLOTHING ARE REQUIRED IN THIS AREA

Employers must ensure that employees who work in or around regulated areas understand the warning signs. Comprehension may necessitate the use of foreign languages, pictographs, and graphics.

At the entrance to mechanical rooms/areas that contain ACM and/or PACM and that employees reasonably can be expected to enter, the building owner is required to post signs that identify the material present, its location, and appropriate work practices that will ensure that ACM and/or PACM will not be disturbed. The employer is required to ensure, to the extent feasible, that employees who come in contact with these signs can comprehend them. Comprehension may necessitate the use of foreign languages, pictographs, graphics, and awareness training. According to OSHA, the standard allows each employer flexibility in deciding how to best ensure that employees in its workplace understand the message conveyed by required warnings.

Warning labels must be put on all products that contain asbestos fibers and their containers. The labels must comply with OSHA's hazard communication standard and include the following information:

DANGER
CONTAINS ASBESTOS FIBERS
AVOID CREATING DUST
CANCER AND LUNG DISEASE HAZARD

Training

Under the construction-activities standard, the employer must set up a training program for all employees who are likely to be exposed in excess of PELs and for all employees who perform Class I through IV asbestos operations.

Employers must ensure employee participation in the program, which must be provided at no cost to employees. Training must be provided prior to or at the time of initial assignment and at least annually thereafter.

Training must cover topics that include

- methods of recognizing asbestos
- health effects associated with asbestos exposure
- the relationship between smoking and asbestos in producing lung cancer
- work operations that can result in exposure
- proper use of respirators
- safe work practices
- medical surveillance requirements

Each class of asbestos work also has its own detailed set of training requirements. For example, training for employees who perform

- Class I operations and for Class II operations that require the use of critical barriers and/or negative-pressure enclosures must be equivalent to the EPA Model Accreditation Plan for asbestos-abatement worker training detailed in 40 CFR 763

- Class IV operations must be consistent with EPA requirements for training of local education agency maintenance and custodial staff as described in 40 CFR 763

Each course must include available information about the location of thermal system insulation, surfacing ACM/PACM, and asbestos-containing flooring material (or flooring material where the absence of asbestos has not been certified) and about instruction in recognition of damage, deterioration, and delamination of asbestos-containing building materials.

A complete list of training requirements is detailed in the standard. The employer must keep all training records for one year beyond the last date of employment.

Medical surveillance

The employer must institute a medical-surveillance program for all employees who, for a combined total of 30 or more days per year, are either of the following:

- Engaged in Class I, II, or III work
- Exposed at or above a PEL (regardless of the type of work performed)

In calculating such exposure, employers need not count any day in which a worker engages in Class II and/or Class III operations on intact material for one hour or less (including cleanup time) and, while doing so, adheres fully to the work practices required by the standard.

Medical-surveillance provisions also require the employer to

- ensure, under the supervision of a physician, that employees who wear negative-pressure respirators are physically able to perform the work and use the equipment
- ensure that all medical examinations and procedures are performed by or under the supervision of a licensed physician, free of charge, and at a reasonable time and place
- establish an accurate record for each employee subject to medical surveillance and keep the record for the duration of employment plus 30 years

Housekeeping

Where vacuuming methods are selected, HEPA-filtered vacuuming equipment must be used and emptied in a manner that minimizes reentry of asbestos into the workplace. Asbestos waste, equipment, and contaminated clothing should be collected and disposed of in sealed, labeled, impermeable bags or containers.

Asbestos-containing flooring material

The following provisions apply to the care of all vinyl and asphalt flooring material, unless the building/facility owner demonstrates that the flooring does not contain asbestos:

- Sanding of flooring material is prohibited
- Stripping of finishes should be conducted using wet methods and low-abrasion pads at speeds lower than 300 revolutions per minute
- Burnishing or dry buffing may be performed only on flooring with sufficient finish to prevent the pad from contacting the flooring material

Waste, debris, and accompanying dust in an area that contains accessible thermal-system insulation, surfacing ACM/PACM, or visibly deteriorated ACM may not be dusted, swept dry, or vacuumed without using a HEPA filter. Such dust and debris should be promptly cleaned up and disposed of in leak-tight containers.

General recordkeeping requirements

OSHA asbestos-exposure standards for both general industry and construction activities require certain records. Records of personal and environmental monitoring for asbestos must be kept for at least 30 years. Records of employees' medical examinations must be kept for the duration of employment plus 30 years.

Exposure records must include

- date of measurement
- operation that involves exposure
- sampling and analytical methods used and evidence of their accuracy
- number, duration, and results of samples taken
- type of respiratory protective devices worn, if any
- name, Social Security number, and exposure of the employee whose exposures are represented

These records must be made available to employees or their designated representatives upon request, and employees must be notified within 15 working days of any exposures that are in excess of the PEL set by OSHA.

Objective data

When the employer has relied on objective data to demonstrate that a certain operation will not expose employees to airborne asbestos fibers at or above the action level, thereby gaining exemption from certain monitoring requirements, an accurate record of the data must be kept to support the exemption.

OSHA permits the employer to utilize the services of competent organizations such as industry trade associations and employee associations to maintain these records. However, the record must include the source of the objective data and other items specified in the regulation.

Medical surveillance

Medical surveillance records must include the name and Social Security number of the employee; medical examination results, including physician recommendations; physician's written opinions, any employee medical complaint related to exposure; and a copy of required information provided to the physician.

Training

All training records must be retained for one year after termination date of an employee.

Record availability

All required exposure and medical records must be made available to OSHA, affected employees, former employees, and designated employee representatives for examination and copying, in accordance with 29 CFR 1910.20.

Transfer of records

When an employer ceases to do business, the employer must transfer all required records to the successor, who must receive and maintain the records. If there is no successor, the employer must notify employees of their rights to access to records at least 90 days prior to close of business and notify NIOSH at least 90 days prior to close of business or disposal of records and transfer the records to NIOSH, upon request.

Records on location of ACM and PACM

The standard for construction activities requires that where building owners and employers use data to demonstrate that PACM does not contain asbestos, such data must be maintained for as long as relied upon to rebut the presumption.

Building owners are required to maintain written records of communication and information they have given or received concerning the identification, location, and quantity of ACM and PACM. Such records must be maintained for the duration of building ownership and must be transferred to successive owners.

Table 1

Respiratory protection for asbestos fibers: General industry

Airborne concentration of asbestos or conditions of use	Required respirator
Not in excess of 1 f/cc (10 x PEL)	Half-mask air-purifying respirator, other than a disposable respirator, equipped with high-efficiency filters.
Not in excess of 5 f/cc (50 x PEL)	Full facepiece air-purifying respirator equipped with high-efficiency filters.
Not in excess of 10 f/cc (100 x PEL)	1. Any powered air-purifying respirator equipped with high-efficiency filters. 2. Any supplied-air respirator operated in continuous-flow mode.
Not in excess of 100 f/cc (1,000 x PEL)	Full facepiece supplied-air respirator operated in pressure-demand mode.
Greater than 100 f/cc (1,000 x PEL) or unknown concentration	Full facepiece supplied-air respirator operated in pressure-demand mode equipped with an auxiliary positive-pressure SCBA.

Note the following:

- Respirators assigned for higher environmental concentrations may be used at lower concentrations.
- A high-efficiency filter means a filter that is at least 99.97% efficient against mono-dispersed particles of 0.3 micrometers or larger.

Table 2

Frequency of chest roentgenograms

Years since first exposure	Age of employee		
	15–35	35–45	45+
0–10	Every five years	Every five years	Every five years
10+	Every five years	Every two years	Every one year

Table 3

Respiratory protection for asbestos fibers: Construction

Airborne concentration of asbestos or conditions of use	Required respirator
Not in excess of 1 f/cc (10 x PEL) or otherwise as required independent of exposure	Half-mask air-purifying respirator, other than a disposable respirator, equipped with high-efficiency filters.
Not in excess of 5 f/cc (50 x PEL)	Full-facepiece air-purifying respirator equipped with high-efficiency filters.
Not in excess of 10 f/cc (100 x PEL)	1. Any PAPR equipped with high-efficiency filters. 2. Any supplied-air respirator operated in continuous-flow mode.
Not in excess of 100 f/cc (1,000 x PEL) or unknown concentration	Full-facepiece supplied-air respirator operated in pressure-demand mode.
Greater than 100 f/cc (1,000 x PEL) or unknown concentration	Full-facepiece supplied-air respirator operated in pressure-demand mode equipped with an auxiliary positive-pressure SCBA.

Note the following:

- Respirators assigned for higher environmental concentrations may be used at lower concentrations; the same applies when required respirator use is independent of concentration.
- A high-efficiency filter means a filter that is at least 99.97% efficient against mono-dispersed particles of 0.3 micrometers or larger.

Bloodborne pathogens (1910.1030)

at a glance

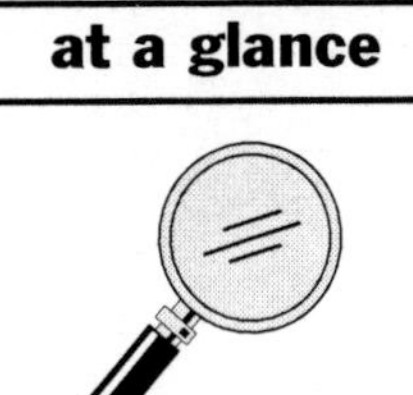

The bloodborne pathogens standard requires various steps and policies for protecting workers from exposure to bloodborne diseases and explains how to report needlestick injuries. During the period October 2003 through September 2004, the bloodborne pathogens standard was the most frequently cited OSHA standard for medical laboratories.

The bloodborne-pathogens standard was issued by OSHA to protect laboratory workers and other employees from on-the-job exposure to diseases transmitted via contact with human blood, blood products, and OPIM such as body fluids, tissues, and virus cultures. The standard was developed primarily to prevent occupational exposure to HBV and HIV. Employees whose work duties are such that they may reasonably be expected to come into contact with blood, blood products, or OPIM are entitled to the protections mandated by the standard.

Employers who fail to comply with the rule may be subject to fines and other penalties authorized by OSHA.

Universal precautions (UPs)

The bloodborne-pathogens standard requires covered employees to observe UPs to prevent exposure to human blood and OPIM. UPs require that all human blood, blood products, and OPIM be treated as though they are known to be infectious, regardless of whether the substance is perceived as coming from a low-risk or high-risk patient or patient group. The UP system relies primarily on the use of gloves and other PPE to prevent exposure to blood and OPIM.

Since the bloodborne-pathogens standard was promulgated, two alternatives to UPs have come into widespread use: BSI and standard precautions. Both systems require laboratory workers to wear gloves and other PPE to prevent exposure to virtually all body substances, mucous membranes, and nonintact skin. This eliminates the need for workers to distinguish between infectious and noninfectious substances when deciding whether to use barrier precautions.

BSI is an acceptable substitute for UPs as long as the employer complies with all other provisions of the standard, according to OSHA's bloodborne-pathogens compliance directive.

Other potentially infectious material (OPIM)

OPIM, as defined in the bloodborne-pathogens standard, includes semen, vaginal secretions, cerebrospinal fluid, synovial fluid, pleural fluid, pericardial fluid, peritoneal fluid, amniotic fluid, saliva in dental procedures, and any body fluid that is visibly contaminated with blood.

OPIM also includes any unfixed tissue or organ (other than intact skin) from a human being who is living or dead; HIV-containing cell or tissue cultures, organ cultures, and HIV- or HBV-containing culture media or other solutions; and blood, organs, or other tissues from experimental animals infected with HIV or HBV.

All body fluids must be treated as potentially infectious in cases where it is difficult or impossible to differentiate between them.

Written exposure-control plan

Establishment of a written exposure-control plan is required for laboratory employers covered by the bloodborne-pathogens standard. The plan generally must identify workers with reasonably anticipated exposure to bloodborne pathogens and specify how those workers will be protected from exposure and trained in prevention methods.

The written plan must include a list of those jobs in which all assigned workers may be exposed to blood or OPIM. It also must contain a list of those jobs in which only some employees are at risk of exposure and a list of those tasks and procedures in which exposures occur for those jobs.

The written plan must be reviewed and updated at least annually and when any new or modified tasks might affect employee exposure. The plan must reflect changes in technology that eliminate or reduce exposure to bloodborne pathogens, and it must document annually the consideration of safer medical devices. Employers must also solicit input from nonmanagement employees who are potentially exposed to sharps injuries. Employee comments on the identification, evaluation, and selection of effective engineering and work-practice controls shall be documented in the exposure control plan. A copy of the plan should be accessible to employees and available for review by OSHA upon request.

Covered employees

The bloodborne-pathogens standard applies to employees who, in the course of performing their jobs, could be exposed to human blood, blood products, or OPIM. Any worker who is subject to health and safety regulations under OSHA's general industry standard (29 CFR 1910) may be covered by the rule. Healthcare-industry employees are the largest group protected by the standard.

Engineering and work-practice controls

OSHA requires employers to reduce or eliminate employee exposure to blood and OPIM through the use of engineering and work-practice controls.

Engineering controls reduce workers' risk of exposure through physical removal or isolation methods. Examples of engineering controls include self-sheathing needles, plastic blood collection tubes, sharps-disposal containers, and safer medical devices, such as needleless systems and sharps with engineered sharps-injury protections.

Work-practice controls reduce exposure risks by altering the manner in which a task is performed, such as through a "no recapping needles" policy.

In cases where exposure potential remains despite use of such controls, PPE also must be used.

Handwashing facilities and practices

Employers must make handwashing facilities available to employees covered by the standard wherever feasible. In other cases, the employer must provide either an appropriate antiseptic hand cleanser, along with clean cloth or paper towels, or antiseptic towelettes until it is possible to wash hands with soap and running water.

Employers are responsible for ensuring that workers wash their hands immediately, or as soon as possible, after removal of gloves or other protective equipment.

The CDC's *Guidelines for Hand Hygiene in Healthcare Settings* (October 2002) further recommend that employees should be offered alcohol-based hand rubs to reduce bacteria. The rubs should not negate the need for soap and water, which continues to be the best practice for removing dirt, blood products, and other visible signs of contamination. Gloves are still recommended for situations where employees have contact with blood or other body fluids, or when they are conducting sterile procedures.

Minimizing exposure to blood and OPIM

To minimize workers' exposure to bloodborne pathogens, the standard specifies the following:

- All procedures that involve blood or OPIM should be performed in a manner that minimizes splashing, spraying, spattering, and generation of droplets. If mucous membranes come into contact with blood, the worker should flush those areas with water immediately or as soon as possible.

- Handling of contact lenses and hand-to-mouth activities, such as eating, drinking, smoking, and applying cosmetics or lip balm, are prohibited in areas where there is a reasonable likelihood of occupational exposure to bloodborne pathogens.

- Food and drink may not be kept in refrigerators, freezers, shelves, or cabinets, or on countertops or benchtops where blood or OPIM are present.
- Mouth pipetting or suctioning of blood or OPIM is prohibited.

Specimens: Containers and handling

Specimens of blood or OPIM must be placed in containers that prevent leakage during collection, handling, processing, storage, transport, or shipping. The container must be closed and either labeled or color-coded prior to being stored, transported, or shipped.

When a facility utilizes UPs in the handling of all specimens, the labeling/color-coding of specimens is not necessary, provided that containers are recognizable as containing specimens. This exemption applies only while the specimen containers remain in the facility.

If the outer surface of the primary container becomes contaminated, it should be placed within a secondary container that prevents leakage and is labeled or color-coded. If the specimen could puncture the primary container, the primary container must be placed in a puncture-resistant secondary container with the above characteristics.

Needles and sharps

Contaminated needles or sharps must not be bent, recapped, or removed from syringes unless the employer can demonstrate that no alternative is feasible or that such action is required by a specific medical procedure. If necessary for that reason, bending, recapping, or removing the needle must be performed using a mechanical device or a one-handed technique. Shearing or breaking of contaminated needles is prohibited.

OSHA further clarified in its compliance directive that blood-tube holders, with needles attached, must be immediately discarded into an accessible sharps container after the safety feature has been activated. The containers also must have an opening that is large enough to accommodate disposal of the entire blood collection assembly (i.e., blood tube holder and needle).

Until properly reprocessed, contaminated reusable sharps must be placed in appropriate containers that are puncture-resistant, labeled or color-coded, and leakproof on the sides and bottom. They must not be stored or processed in a way that requires employees to reach by hand into the containers where the sharps have been placed.

Contaminated sharps must be discarded in closable containers that are puncture-resistant, leakproof on sides and bottom, and labeled or color-coded. During use, containers for contaminated sharps must be easily accessible to personnel and located as close as possible to the immediate area where sharps are used or normally found. These containers must be upright throughout use, replaced routinely, and not allowed to overfill.

When moving containers of contaminated sharps from the area of use, containers must be closed and care must be taken to prevent spills or protrusion of contents. Reusable containers may not be opened, emptied, cleaned by hand, or handled in any manner that could expose employees to the risk of injuring their skin.

Waste disposal

Mechanical means—such as a brush and dustpan, tongs, or forceps—must be used to pick up potentially contaminated broken glassware.

Other regulated waste must be placed in containers that are closable, constructed to contain all contents without protrusion, leakproof, and labeled or color-coded. Containers must be closed prior to removal to prevent spillage during handling, storage, transport, or shipping.

Regulated waste is defined by OSHA as

- liquid or semi-liquid blood or OPIM
- contaminated items that would release blood or OPIM in a liquid or semi-liquid state if compressed
- items that are caked with dried blood or OPIM and are capable of releasing these materials during handling
- contaminated sharps
- pathological and microbiological wastes containing blood or OPIM

All regulated waste disposal must comply with other applicable federal and state regulations.

Housekeeping

The work site must be maintained in a clean and sanitary condition, and employers are required to create/maintain an appropriate written schedule for cleaning and for methods of decontamination. The standard also requires that

- all equipment and working surfaces are cleaned and disinfected after contact with blood or OPIM
- protective coverings such as plastic wrap, aluminum foil, or imperviously backed absorbent paper used to cover equipment and environmental surfaces be removed and replaced as soon as possible after they become contaminated, or at the end of the work shift if they have become contaminated during the shift
- all bins, pails, cans, and similar receptacles intended for reuse be inspected and decontaminated regularly, or cleaned and decontaminated immediately if there is visible contamination

Laundry

Contaminated laundry should be handled as little as possible. It must be bagged or put in containers at the location where it was used, but it cannot be sorted or rinsed in that location. Bags or containers in which the laundry is placed and transported must be labeled or color-coded sufficiently to permit all employees to recognize the containers as having contaminated contents.

When contaminated laundry is wet, it must be placed and transported in bags or containers that prevent soak-through or leakage to the exterior.

Appropriate PPE, such as gloves, must be worn by employees who have contact with contaminated laundry. It is the employer's responsibility to ensure that workers comply with this requirement.

Equipment cleaning and servicing

Equipment that may become contaminated with blood or OPIM must be examined prior to servicing or shipping and must be decontaminated if possible. A label must be attached to the equipment that states which portions remain contaminated, and the employer must ensure that this information is conveyed to all affected employees, the servicing representative, and/or the manufacturer prior to handling, servicing, or shipping so that appropriate precautions can be taken.

PPE

When there is potential for occupational exposure to bloodborne pathogens, employers must provide PPE for employees at no cost. Such equipment includes but is not limited to items such as gloves, gowns, laboratory coats, face shields or masks, eye protection, and ventilation devices such as mouthpieces, resuscitation bags, and pocket masks.

PPE is adequate only if it does not permit blood or OPIM to pass through to or reach the employee's work clothes, street clothes, undergarments, skin, eyes, mouth, or other mucous membranes under normal conditions of use and for the duration of time during which the protective equipment will be used.

Use and selection

It is the employer's responsibility to ensure that employees use the appropriate PPE. The only exception to this may be made in cases where the employer can show that an employee declined to use equipment for only a brief time, based on the judgment that its use would have prevented the delivery of services or would have posed an increased safety hazard.

In addition, the employer is responsible for making the PPE readily accessible to employees and providing appropriate sizes. Glove liners, powderless gloves, or other alternatives must be readily accessible to employees who are allergic to the gloves normally provided.

Laundry and disposal

Employers are responsible for cleaning, laundering, and disposing of PPE at no cost to employees. The equipment must be repaired and replaced as needed to maintain its effectiveness. This, too, must be at no cost to the employee.

Garments penetrated by blood or OPIM must be removed immediately or as soon as feasible. All PPE must be removed before leaving the work area.

Gloves

Gloves must be worn when it is reasonably anticipated that the worker may have hand contact with blood, OPIM, mucous membranes, or nonintact skin; when performing vascular access procedures; and when handling or touching contaminated items or surfaces.

Disposable gloves such as surgical or examination gloves must be replaced as soon as practical when contaminated, or as soon as feasible if they are torn, punctured, or when their ability to provide an effective barrier is lost. These gloves should not be washed or decontaminated for reuse.

Utility gloves may be decontaminated for reuse if the integrity of the gloves is not compromised. However, they must be discarded if they are cracked, peeling, torn, punctured, or exhibiting other signs of deterioration.

Face and clothing protection

Employees are required to wear masks, eye protection, and face shields whenever there is the possibility that splashes, spray, spatter, or droplets of blood or OPIM could contaminate the eyes, nose, or mouth.

The standard requires employees to wear masks in combination with eye-protection devices, such as goggles or glasses with solid side shields or chin-length face shields.

Gowns, aprons, and other protective clothing also may be required, depending on the task and degree of occupational exposure anticipated. Such items may include gowns, aprons, lab coats, clinic jackets, or similar outer garments.

Surgical caps and hoods and shoe coverings and/or boots must be worn in instances when gross contamination can reasonably be expected.

Vaccination and postexposure follow-up

Employers must make hepatitis B vaccines available to all employees who may be exposed to blood or OPIM on the job. Postexposure follow-up and evaluation also must be made available to those employees who have had an exposure incident.

All of these medical services, including the vaccine and postexposure evaluation and follow-up, must be offered at a reasonable time and place and provided at no cost to the employee. The procedures must be performed by or under the supervision of a physician or other licensed healthcare professional. Laboratory tests should be conducted by an accredited laboratory. All medical evaluations and procedures should be provided according to current recommendations of the U.S. Public Health Service.

Employees who choose not to be vaccinated must sign a declination form that attests to the fact that they have been offered the vaccine and that they understand their risk of occupational exposure. The form must contain language specified by OSHA.

Vaccination procedures

The hepatitis B vaccination should be made available after the employee has received information that concerns its safety and purpose and within 10 working days of initial assignment. Exceptions are allowed in cases where the employee already has received the complete vaccination series, has been shown through antibody testing to be immune to the virus, or cannot take the vaccine because of medical reasons. Employers may not make participation in a prescreening program a prerequisite for receiving the hepatitis B vaccination.

Postexposure testing

Following a report of an exposure incident, the employer is required to immediately offer the exposed employee (at no charge) a confidential medical evaluation and follow-up. At a minimum, they should include the following elements:

- Documentation of the route(s) of exposure and the circumstances under which the exposure incident occurred.

- Identification and documentation of the source individual, unless the employer can establish that identification is infeasible or prohibited by state law.

- Testing of the employee's blood for HBV/HIV as soon as possible after consent is obtained. If the employee consents to baseline blood collection, but does not give consent at that time for HIV serologic testing, the sample should be preserved for 90 days. If, within that time, the employee elects to have the baseline sample tested, such testing must be done as soon as possible.

- Postexposure prophylaxis, when medically indicated.

- Counseling.

- Evaluation of reported illnesses.

Information provided to the healthcare professional

The following information must be provided to the healthcare professional who is responsible for an employee's hepatitis B vaccination:

- A copy of the bloodborne pathogens standard
- A description of the exposed employee's duties as they relate to the exposure incident
- Documentation of the routes of exposure and the circumstances under which the exposure occurred
- Results of the source individual's blood testing, if available
- All medical records relevant to the appropriate treatment of the employee, including vaccination status, which are the employer's responsibility to maintain

Written medical evaluation

The employer must provide the employee with a copy of the evaluating healthcare professional's written opinion within 15 days of the completion of the evaluation.

The written opinion for hepatitis B vaccination should be limited to stating whether the vaccination is indicated for the employee and whether the employee has received the vaccination.

The healthcare professional's written opinion for postexposure evaluation and follow-up should state only that the employee was informed of the results of the evaluation and that the employee was told about any medical conditions resulting from exposure to blood or OPIM that require further evaluation or treatment.

All other findings or diagnoses must be kept confidential and may not be included in the written report.

Hepatitis B vaccine for first-aid providers

First-aid providers whose primary job is not first-aid administration (e.g., office employees who are trained in first-aid techniques) do not necessarily have to be offered a preexposure hepatitis B vaccine under the bloodborne pathogens rule, according to an OSHA compliance directive. The agency said failure to provide such employees with the vaccine would be considered a de minimis violation and would not result in a citation as long as the following conditions are met:

- The designated first-aid provider's primary job is not the rendering of first aid.
- The full hepatitis B vaccination series is offered to all unvaccinated first-aid providers in a situation where blood or OPIM was present, regardless of whether a specific exposure incident has occurred. The vaccine must be provided as soon as possible and within 24 hours.
- All first-aid incidents that involve blood or OPIM are reported to the employer before the end of the work shift. The report must include the names of all first-aid providers who rendered assistance, a description of the incident, and a determination of whether an actual exposure incident occurred. The report must be recorded on a list of such first-aid incidents and must be readily available to all employees and to OSHA upon request.
- A bloodborne-pathogens training program that includes the specifics of the reporting procedure is provided to all designated first-aid providers.
- The employer's written exposure-control plan describes the first-aid policy and reporting procedures.

If the first-aid provider responds to an emergency in which blood or OPIM are present, the employer must provide the HBV vaccine and comply with other postexposure follow-up requirements.

The exemption does not apply to first-aid providers who give assistance on a regular basis, such as at a first-aid station, clinic, or other location where injured employees routinely go for treatment. These employees and other healthcare, emergency, and public safety personnel whose job duties regularly include provision of first aid remain fully covered by the standard and must be offered a preexposure vaccine.

Research laboratories and production facilities

Additional precautions must be taken to protect employees in research laboratories and production facilities engaged in the culture, production, concentration, experimentation, and manipulation of HIV and HBV. These additional requirements do not apply to clinical or diagnostic laboratories engaged solely in the analysis of blood, tissues, or organs.

Biosafety manual

A biosafety manual must be prepared or adopted and periodically reviewed. It must be updated at least annually or as often as necessary.

Decontamination and waste handling

OSHA requires that research laboratories and production facilities follow standard microbiological practices and incinerate or decontaminate all regulated waste by a method that is known to effectively destroy bloodborne pathogens (e.g., autoclaving).

In addition, the standard requires that all waste from work areas and from animal rooms must either be incinerated or decontaminated by a method such as autoclaving before disposal.

Contaminated materials that are to be decontaminated at a site away from the work area must be placed in a durable, leakproof, and labeled or color-coded container that is closed before being removed from the work area.

Restricted access

Production facilities and research laboratories must establish written policies and procedures to ensure that access to the work area is limited to authorized persons. Such persons must be advised of the potential biohazard, meet specific entry requirements, and comply with entry and exit procedures.

Laboratory doors must be kept closed when work that involves HIV or HBV is in progress. A hazard warning sign must be posted on all access doors whenever potentially infectious materials or infected animals are present in the work area or containment module. The sign must incorporate the universal BIOHAZARD symbol.

PPE

Appropriate protective clothing must be worn in the work area and animal rooms. This may include laboratory coats, gowns, smocks, or uniforms.

Protective clothing must not be worn outside of the work area and must be decontaminated before laundering. Gloves must be worn when handling infected animals and when making hand contact with OPIM. Special care must be taken to avoid skin contact.

Vacuum lines must be protected with liquid-disinfectant traps and HEPA filters, or filters of equivalent or superior efficiency. The filters must be checked routinely and maintained or replaced as necessary.

Restricted use of needles

To reduce the risk of exposure through needlestick injuries, research-laboratory and production-facility workers may use hypodermic needles and syringes only for parenteral injection and aspiration of fluids from laboratory animals and diaphragm bottles.

Only needle-locking syringes may be used for the injection and aspiration of OPIM. Extreme caution must be used when handling needles and syringes. A needle may not be bent, sheared, replaced in the sheath or guard, or removed from the syringe following use.

The standard requires that the needle and syringe promptly be placed in a puncture-resistant container and autoclaved or decontaminated before reuse or disposal.

Spills

The standard requires that all spills be contained immediately and cleaned up by appropriate professional staff or others properly trained or equipped to work with potentially infectious materials. A spill or accident that results in an exposure incident must immediately be reported to the laboratory director or other responsible person.

Containment modules and safety cabinets

No work with OPIM is permitted on the open bench. The work must be conducted in biological safety cabinets or other physical containment devices within the containment module.

Certified biological safety cabinets (Class I, II, or III) or other combinations of personal protection or physical containment devices must be used for all activities with OPIM that pose a threat of exposure to droplets, splashes, spills, or aerosols. The standard requires biological safety cabinets to be certified when installed, whenever they are moved, and at least annually.

Research labs: Other requirements

Research laboratories must have a facility for hand- and eye-washing readily available in each laboratory, as well as an autoclave for decontaminated waste.

Production facilities: Other requirements

HIV and HBV production facilities must meet the following criteria:

- Two sets of doors must be used for passage into the work area from access corridors or other contiguous areas.

- Surfaces of doors, walls, floors, and ceilings in the work area must be water-resistant so they can be easily cleaned. Penetrations in the surfaces must be sealed or capable of being sealed to simplify decontamination.

- Each work area must have a sink for washing hands and a readily accessible facility for eye washing. The sink must be foot-, elbow-, or automatically operated and must be located near the exit door of the work area.

- An autoclave for decontamination of regulated waste must be available within or as near as possible to the work area.

- Access doors to the work area or containment module must be self-closing.

- A ducted exhaust-air ventilation system must be provided to create directional airflow that draws air into the work area through the entry area. The exhaust air must not be recirculated to any other area of the building, must be discharged to the outside, and must be dispersed away from occupied areas and air intake. The proper direction of the airflow must be verified.

Information and training

Employers are required to provide all employees who are covered under the bloodborne-pathogens standard with training that meets the program requirements described in this section. The training must be provided to full-time, part-time, and temporary employees during working hours and at no cost to the worker.

Training material should be appropriate in content and vocabulary to the education level, literacy, and language of employees.

Training frequency

Employers are required under the standard to provide training to covered employees at the time of initial assignment to tasks where occupational exposure to blood or OPIM may take place and at least annually thereafter. Annual training for all employees must be provided within one year of their previous training.

Additional training is required when changes to tasks or procedures take place or when new tasks and procedures are introduced. The additional training need only include information about the new exposures created.

Minimum program requirements

At a minimum, the employer's training program must provide an accessible copy of the text of the bloodborne-pathogens standard and an explanation of its contents. The program also must contain the following:

- An explanation of the epidemiology and symptoms of bloodborne diseases and their modes of transmission
- An explanation of the employer's written exposure-control plan and the means by which employees may obtain copies
- Instruction on how to recognize tasks and other activities that may involve exposure to blood and OPIM
- An explanation of the use and limitations of methods that will prevent or reduce exposure, including appropriate engineering controls, work practices, and PPE
- Information about the types, proper use, location, removal, handling, decontamination, and disposal of PPE
- An explanation of the basis for selection of PPE
- Information about the hepatitis B vaccine, including its effectiveness and safety, method of administration, the benefits of being vaccinated, and a statement that the vaccine and vaccination are offered free of charge
- Information about the appropriate actions to take and the persons to contact in an emergency that involves blood or OPIM
- An explanation of the procedure to follow if an exposure incident occurs, including the method of reporting the incident and the medical follow-up to be made available

- Information about the postexposure evaluation and follow-up that must be provided following an exposure incident

- An explanation of the signs and labels and/or color-coding required by the standard

Employees must have an opportunity to ask questions during and/or after the training session.

Trainer qualifications

The standard specifies that the person who conducts the required training must be knowledgeable both in the general subject matter and in its application to the workplace at hand.

Examples of qualified trainers would include infection-control practitioners, nurse practitioners, and registered nurses. Examples of qualified nonhealthcare professionals include industrial hygienists, epidemiologists, and professional trainers, provided that they can demonstrate evidence of specialized training in the area of bloodborne pathogens.

Research laboratories and production facilities: Additional training

Employees in HIV and HBV laboratories and production facilities must receive further training in addition to the above training requirements.

The employer must ensure that these employees

- demonstrate proficiency in standard microbiological practices and techniques and in the practices and operations specific to the facility before they are allowed to work with HIV or HBV

- have prior experience in the handling of human pathogens or tissue cultures before working with HIV or HBV

- participate in work activities only after proficiency has been demonstrated

Employees without prior experience handling human pathogens must be provided with appropriate training. Such employees' initial work assignments may not include the handling of infectious agents. Rather, a progression of work activities should be assigned as techniques are learned and proficiency developed. The employer must ensure that employees participate in work activities involving infectious agents only after they demonstrate proficiency in doing so.

Warning labels

Warning labels must be affixed to containers of regulated waste, refrigerators and freezers that contain blood or OPIM, and other containers used to store, transport, or ship blood or OPIM.

Exemptions to this provision are allowed for the following:

- Red bags or containers that are substituted for labels
- Containers of blood, blood components, or blood products that are labeled as to their contents and have been released for transfusion or other clinical use
- Individual containers of blood or OPIM that are placed in a labeled container during storage, transport, shipment, or disposal

Regulated waste that has been decontaminated does not have to be labeled or color-coded.

Required labels should be affixed as close as possible to the container by string, wire, adhesive, or another method that prevents their loss or unintentional removal.

Labels required for contaminated equipment must state which portions of the equipment remain contaminated.

The BIOHAZARD symbol must be included on all labels required under the standard. The symbol must be fluorescent orange/orange-red or predominantly so, with lettering and symbols in a contrasting color.

Sign posting

Warning signs must be posted at the entrance to work areas in HIV and HBV research laboratories and production facilities. Signs must bear the BIOHAZARD symbol with the name of the infectious agent, special requirements for entering the area, and the name and telephone number of the laboratory director or other responsible person. These signs must be fluorescent orange-red or predominantly so, with lettering and symbols in a contrasting color.

Recordkeeping

Medical records

The bloodborne-pathogens standard requires that an accurate medical record be maintained for each covered employee. The medical records should be maintained in compliance with OSHA's rules on employee access and transfer of records (see Access to records chapter).

Under the bloodborne-pathogens standard, the record must contain the following:

- The name and Social Security number of the employee
- A copy of the employee's hepatitis B status, including the dates of all hepatitis B vaccinations and any medical records relative to the employee's ability to receive vaccination
- A copy of all results of any postexposure medical evaluation and follow-up procedures
- A copy of the healthcare professional's written opinion
- A copy of the information provided to the healthcare professional, if applicable

Medical records must be kept confidential and not disclosed or reported without the employee's written consent to any person within or outside the workplace except as required by law. The records must be maintained for at least the duration of employment plus 30 years. All required records must be made available to OSHA if the agency requests them.

Training records

Training records required under the standard must include the following:

- Dates of training sessions
- Contents and summary of the training sessions
- Names and qualifications of persons who conduct the training
- Names and job titles of all persons who attend the training sessions

Training records should be maintained for three years from the date on which the training occurred. Training records must be provided upon request for examination and copying to the individuals they pertain to, their representatives (e.g., union stewards), and OSHA.

Sharps injury log

Employers are required to establish and maintain a sharps injury log for recording percutaneous injuries from contaminated sharps. The information in the sharps injury log must be recorded and maintained in such manner as to protect the confidentiality of the injured employee.

The sharps injury log must contain the following:

- The type and brand of device involved in the incident
- The department or work area where the exposure incident occurred
- An explanation of how the incident occurred

Compressed gases (1910.169)

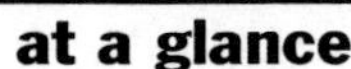

at a glance

OSHA incorporates standards from other organizations for the storage, handling, and use of compressed gases.

Compressed gases used in laboratories include nitrogen (gas and liquid), carbon dioxide, and hydrogen. Some laboratories may also use acetylene, oxygen, and some inert gases such as helium or argon. Liquid CO_2 may also be used as a refrigerant, usually as a backup in ultra-low freezers. Depending on the reason for use, some laboratories use various mixtures of gases, especially carbon dioxide and nitrogen.

Compressed gases can be combustible, flammable, explosive, poisonous, and/or corrosive. Because some compressed gases are flammable and all cylinders are under pressure, they must be handled with extreme care. An exploding cylinder can have the same effect as a bomb.

All handling, storage, and utilization of compressed gases must be in accordance with standards issued by the CGA. OSHA requirements are listed in the compressed gas and compressed-air standards (Subpart M—29 CFR 1910.169–171). The OSHA standard incorporates by reference certain standards developed by the CGA, the ASME, the NFPA, and ANSI.

Handling

The proper handling of compressed gas cylinders requires training and a well-enforced safety program. All laboratory employees who handle gas should be familiar not only with the physiological effects but also with the control measures. Although it is the employee's obligation to adhere strictly to the safety standards, it is management's obligation to train the workers thoroughly.

The greatest care should be exercised in the handling of cylinders. They should never collide or be dropped. Nothing should be allowed to fall on them.

Most cylinders have a steel protective cap that screws on over the valve. Except when cylinders are in use, the caps should remain screwed down to the last thread. When cylinders are moved, special hand trucks should be used. When in transit, the cylinders should be lashed to the cradles of the trucks in as near to an upright position as possible.

OSHA requires employers to ensure that unloading operations are performed by reliable persons who are properly instructed in doing so. Employees should know the chemical and physical hazards with which they work, and must be thoroughly familiar with the types of PPE provided for their safety. They also should be instructed in first-aid procedures.

Improper handling of compressed-gas cylinders can produce a hazard called "rocketing." If an accidental rupture occurs, or if a valve assembly is snapped off, such a cylinder can blast through a concrete wall.

Storage

Compressed-gas cylinders should be examined for damage and leaks as soon as they are received. If there are any signs of damage or leakage, they should be moved to a safe, isolated area and returned to the supplier as soon as possible.

Cylinders must be stored upright in a safe, dry, well-ventilated area, away from any source of heat and away from electrical wiring. Storage areas must be fire-resistant, clean, free of combustible materials, and well-lighted. Cylinders must be secured in an upright position by chain, cable, or other suitable means to prevent tumbling.

Compressed-gas cylinders should never be subjected to temperatures higher than 125° F.

Cylinders should not be stored near steam pipes, hot-water pipes, boilers, highly flammable solvents, combustible wastes, unprotected electrical connections, open flames, or other potential sources of heat or ignition. Cylinders should be properly labeled. The valve-protection cap should not be removed until the cylinder is secured and ready for use. Cylinders of oxygen may not be stored near cylinders that contain flammable gases. Empty cylinders are required to be marked "EMPTY" and kept away from full ones. Full cylinders must be positively identified as to the gases they contain.

Compressed air

Misuse of compressed-air equipment that results in injury to employees can be reduced with proper training. Employees should be familiar with the air compressor's operating and maintenance instructions.

Compressed air may not be used for cleaning purposes under OSHA regulations for hand-held tools (OSHA Standards Subpart P—29 CFR 1910.242[b]), unless pressure is reduced to less than 30 psi and effective chip-guarding and PPE are used. An OSHA directive (OSHA Instruction STD 1-13.1, October 1978) provides guidance and examples of what alternative systems may be used to meet these requirements. According to OSHA, "reduce to less than 30 psi" means that the downstream pressure of the air at the nozzle (nozzle pressure) or opening of a gun, pipe, cleaning lance, etc., used for cleaning purposes should remain at a pressure level below 30 psi for all static conditions. "Effective chip-guarding" refers to any method or equipment that will prevent a chip or particle from being blown into the eyes or unbroken skin of the operator of cleaning equipment or other workers.

OSHA also requires the following:

- New air tanks must be constructed in accordance with appropriate sections of the ASME Boiler and Pressure Vessel Code. The code requires this information to be stamped permanently on the air tank.

- The drain valve on the air tank should be opened frequently to prevent excessive accumulation of liquid.

- Air tanks must be protected by adequate safety relief valve(s). These valves must be tested at regular intervals to be sure they are in good operating condition.

- The pressure controller and gauge must be maintained in good operating condition.
- There should not be valves between the air tank and the safety valve.

Carbon dioxide

Carbon dioxide, which is odorless, colorless, and heavier than air, is toxic when high percentages are present and can cause death when encountered in asphyxiating concentrations. This gas is not flammable and is in common use as a fire-extinguishing agent. Because of its ability to displace oxygen, it will smother the fires of petroleum, coal, and wood; however, the fires of magnesium, sodium, potassium, and metal hydrides will burn rapidly in an atmosphere of carbon dioxide.

Hydrogen

Hydrogen, the lightest of all elements, is colorless and odorless. Its flammable range is almost as wide as that of acetylene. A mixture of 10%–65% in air will explode if ignited. Hydrogen is classified as an asphyxiant.

Some chemical reactions produce hydrogen as a byproduct. A lead-acid battery will produce hydrogen when charged. Many electroplating processes also produce hydrogen. Some chemicals used to remove scale from the waterside of boilers manufacture hydrogen. Whatever the operation, it is important to know whether hydrogen will be produced, and measures must be taken to prevent its accumulation and ignition. This is accomplished by proper ventilation and elimination of possible sources of ignition.

Storing hydrogen is difficult. This gas tries to find its way out of confinement and will seek the smallest opening in a pipe or container. Pipe threads and stems must be tight because a high-pressure hydrogen leak can ignite spontaneously from the friction of its own escape. All flammable gas leaks are dangerous, particularly when, as in the case of hydrogen, they can be neither seen nor smelled.

Oxygen

Although oxygen supports combustion, it does not burn. Oxygen is considered a hazardous element because flammable materials burn much more quickly in oxygen, and oxygen can combine quickly with other elements and compounds to produce spontaneous ignition. When oxygen comes into contact with oil, grease, or fuel oils, the result can be a sudden and violent fire. Employees involved in the handling of this gas must take every precaution to prevent the combination. Liquid oxygen can be equally dangerous if not handled properly. A burning cigarette dropped into liquid oxygen will produce a flame two feet high, and even shredded metal will burn if exposed to it. Open flames and smoking must never be allowed near oxygen storage areas.

Confined spaces (1910.146)

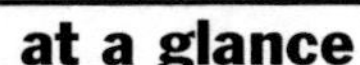

at a glance

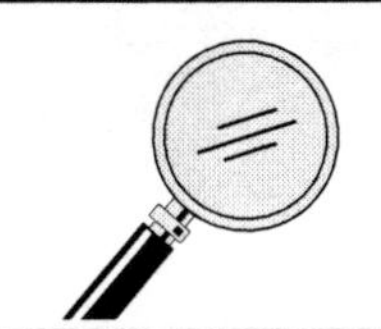

The confined-space standard sets requirements for employees entering confined spaces (areas into which a person can fit but which have limited exit and entry points, such as a vault).

OSHA's permit-required confined-space standard (29 CFR 1910.146) covers all of general industry, including laboratories. The standard applies to boilers, storage vessels, furnaces, railroad tank cars, manholes, and cooking and process vessels, among other spaces.

The standard is intended to protect workers from toxic, explosive, or asphyxiating atmospheres and from possible engulfment by small particles, such as grain or sawdust. It focuses on areas with immediate health or safety risks, denoting them as "permit-required" confined spaces.

Employers are required by the rule to identify all permit-required spaces in their workplaces, prevent unauthorized entry into them, and protect authorized workers from hazards through a permit-space program.

The permit-space program should include

- identification and control of hazards
- entry procedures
- appropriate training and equipment for authorized entrants, entry supervisors, and attendants
- documented compliance through written permits
- attendants to control or monitor entry operations

The standard also mandates advance planning, appropriate precautions for rescuing entrants, and coordination with contractors involved in confined-space entry. If the sole risk to workers is a hazardous atmosphere that can be eliminated through forced air ventilation, attendants would not be required as long as strict entry procedures are followed.

OSHA amended the confined-space standard to ensure employee involvement in the development and implementation of permit-space programs, allow authorized permit-space entrants or their authorized representatives the opportunity to observe any testing or monitoring of permit spaces, and clarify requirements related to preparation for rescues from confined spaces.

The standard has six appendices. These include a decision flow chart for determining whether a confined space will require an entry permit, procedures for atmospheric testing, model permit-required space programs, sample permits, a representative program for sewer-system safety, and evaluation criteria for selecting a rescue team or rescue service.

Violations of the confined-space rule generally will be classified as serious because of the danger of death or serious injury to an employee.

Applicability

The standard covers general industry workers, including 1.6 million who enter confined spaces annually and an additional 10.6 million employed at the 240,000 work sites covered by the standard (29 CFR 1910.146[a]).

"Confined space" is defined as an area that

- has adequate size and configuration for employee entry
- has limited means of access or egress
- is not designed for continuous employee occupancy

The standard defines a permit-required confined space as a confined space that has one or more of the following characteristics:

- Contains or has the potential to contain a hazardous atmosphere

- Contains a material that has the potential for engulfing an entrant

- Has an internal configuration such that the entrant could be trapped or asphyxiated by inwardly converging walls or by a floor that slopes downward and tapers to a smaller cross-section

- Contains any other serious safety or health hazard

The definition of "confined space" generally is limited to areas where an employee must enter or exit in a posture that might slow self-rescue or make rescue more difficult, such as a manhole or a hatch in a storage tank. However, OSHA has clarified that for the purposes of this regulation, a confined space may include areas that have a door or portal through which a person can walk upright when the door or portal is obstructed in a way that hinders the entrant's ability to escape in an emergency.

A prohibited condition is defined as any condition not allowed by permit during entry operations.

Confined spaces in laboratories

Many spaces in laboratory facilities may fit OSHA's definition of confined space. It can be difficult to determine which of those spaces are permit-required and which are not. Often, the decision must be made on a case-by-case basis.

The key to defining a permit-required space centers around the degree of hazard presented to an employee who works in the space, taking into consideration both the type of space and the work to be done. The greater the hazard, the more likely the space would be considered permit-required. If an obviously grave danger exists, it is highly likely that the space is permit-required.

Permit-required confined spaces that may be present in laboratory facilities include boilers, sterilizers, ventilation systems, or underground storage tanks. Other confined spaces, which may or may not qualify as permit-required depending on the work to be done, might include interstitial areas between walls and manholes or pits on facility grounds.

Work-site evaluation

The standard requires employers initially to evaluate their workplaces and determine whether there are any permit-required confined spaces. If the workplace contains permit spaces, the employer must inform employees by posting danger signs, or any other equally effective warning, to alert employees to the existence, location, and danger posed by the permit spaces.

Permit-required confined-space program

The standard requires employers to establish a written program to prevent unauthorized entry, identify and evaluate hazards, and establish procedures and practices for safe entry, including testing and monitoring conditions.

Employers must consult with affected employees and their authorized representatives on the development and implementation of the permit-space program.

Under the standard, employers must develop means, procedures, and practices for safe permit-space entry that include but are not limited to

- specifying acceptable entry conditions
- providing authorized entrants or their authorized representatives the opportunity to observe any monitoring or testing of permit spaces
- isolating the permit space
- purging, inerting, flushing, or ventilating the permit space as necessary to eliminate or control atmospheric hazards

- providing pedestrian, vehicle, or other necessary barriers to protect entrants from external hazards

- verifying that conditions in the permit space are acceptable for entry throughout the duration of an authorized entry

Employers must, at no cost to employees, provide any equipment necessary for safe entry, maintain such equipment, and ensure its proper use by employees. Such equipment could include

- testing and monitoring equipment
- ventilation equipment needed to ensure acceptable entry conditions
- communications equipment necessary for the safety of entrants in case of emergency
- PPE, if feasible engineering and work-practice controls are not adequate
- lighting equipment
- barriers and shields
- ladders as necessary for safe entrance to and exit from the space
- any necessary rescue equipment
- any other equipment necessary for safe entry into and rescue from permit spaces

Testing and monitoring

The permit-required confined-space program also must include procedures for testing and monitoring the permit space. Conditions in the permit space must be tested to determine whether acceptable entry conditions exist before entry is authorized. Monitoring must continue as necessary to determine whether acceptable entry conditions are maintained during the course of entry operations.

When testing for atmospheric hazards, employers should test first for oxygen, then for combustible gases and vapors, and then for toxic air contaminants, according to the standard.

Authorized entrants or their authorized representatives must be permitted to observe preentry testing and any subsequent testing or monitoring of permit spaces. The employer is required to reevaluate the permit space in the presence of any authorized personnel who question the adequacy of the initial evaluation. The results of any testing must be provided immediately to each authorized entrant or to that employee's authorized representative.

The standard further requires that the permit program include the means and procedures that will enable the attendant to respond to an emergency that affects one or more of the permit spaces being monitored, without distraction from the attendant's responsibilities if multiple spaces are to be monitored by a single attendant.

Personnel roles

The written program also must designate the persons who are to have active roles in entry operations (for example, authorized entrants, attendants, entry supervisors, or persons who test or monitor the atmosphere in a permit space), identify the duties of each such employee, and provide each such employee with appropriate training.

The program also calls for an attendant stationed outside permit spaces during entry, procedures to summon rescuers and prevent unauthorized personnel from attempting rescue, and a system for preparing, issuing, using, and canceling entry permits.

The program must include requirements for coordinating entry for more than one employer, procedures for concluding entry operations, and procedures for canceling entry permits.

Program review

A review of the permit-required confined-space program, using the canceled permits required to be maintained, must be performed within one year after each entry. The program must be revised as necessary to ensure that employees who participate in entry operations are protected from permit-space hazards.

Permit system

Before entry is authorized, the employer must document the completion of required safety measures by preparing an entry permit. The standard requires an entry supervisor to authorize entry, prepare and sign written permits, order corrective measures if necessary, and cancel permits when work is completed. The completed permit must be made available at the time of entry to all authorized entrants or their authorized representatives by posting it at the entry portal or by any other equally effective means, so that the entrants can confirm that preentry preparations have been completed.

Permits must not exceed the time required to complete the assigned task or job identified on the permit and must be retained for at least one year to facilitate review of the confined-space program.

Entry permits

Under the confined-space entry standard, entry permits must include

- identification of the confined space
- purpose of the entry
- date and authorized duration of the permit
- list of authorized entrants
- names of current attendants and entry supervisor
- list of hazards in the permit space
- list of measures to isolate permit space and eliminate or control hazards

The permit also must state

- the acceptable entry conditions
- results of tests, initialed by the person or persons performing the tests
- rescue and emergency services to be summoned and the means for summoning those services
- communication procedures used by authorized entrants and attendants to maintain contact during entry

- required equipment (such as respirators, communications, alarm systems, etc.)
- any additional permits, such as for hot work, that have been issued to authorize work in the permit space
- any other information that may be necessary to ensure safety

Training

The standard requires employers to conduct initial training for employees who will enter confined spaces and refresher training for when duties change, hazards in the confined space change, or evaluation determines inadequacies in the employees' knowledge. Training must provide employees with understanding, skills, and knowledge to do the job safely.

Employers must certify that the required training has been accomplished. The certification must contain each employee's name, the signatures or initials of the trainers, and the dates of the training. Training certification must be available for inspection by employees and their authorized representatives.

Authorized entrants

Under the standard, employers must ensure that all authorized entrants to confined spaces

- know the hazards they may face
- are able to recognize signs or symptoms of exposure and understand the consequences of exposure to hazards
- know how to use any needed equipment

- communicate with the attendant as necessary to enable the attendant to both monitor entrant status and alert entrants of the need to evacuate the space if necessary

- alert attendants when a warning symptom or other hazardous condition exists

- exit as quickly as possible whenever ordered or alerted (by alarm, warning sign, or prohibited condition) to do so

Attendants

Specific provisions of the standard require the employer to ensure that each attendant

- knows the hazards of confined spaces and is aware of behavioral effects of potential exposures

- continuously maintains an accurate count of authorized entrants in the permit space and ensures that the means used to identify authorized entrants identifies who is in the permit space

- remains outside the permit space during entry operations until relieved by another attendant

- communicates with authorized entrants in order to monitor entrant status and to alert entrants of the need to evacuate

Attendants also must

- monitor activities inside and outside the permit space and order exit if required
- summon rescuers if necessary
- prevent unauthorized entry into the permit space
- perform nonentry rescues if required

Attendants are not allowed to perform duties that interfere with their primary duty of monitoring and protecting the safety of authorized entrants.

Entry supervisors

The standard requires employers to ensure that entry supervisors

- know the hazards of confined spaces
- verify that all tests have been conducted and all procedures and equipment are in place before endorsing the permit
- terminate entry and cancel permits
- verify that rescue services and the means for summoning them are available
- remove unauthorized individuals who enter or attempt to enter the permit space during entry operations
- determine, at least when shifts and entry supervisors change, that acceptable conditions as specified in the permit are maintained

Rescue and emergency services

Under the standard, employers must develop procedures for summoning rescue and emergency services and for rescuing entrants from permit spaces, when necessary. Employers also must develop procedures to provide necessary emergency services to rescued employees and to prevent unauthorized personnel from attempting a rescue.

Rescue and emergency services may be performed by on-site or off-site rescue personnel.

Off-site services

In selecting off-site rescue teams or services, employers must evaluate the rescuers' ability to make a timely response and function appropriately while rescuing permit-space entrants. The employer must select a rescue team or service from those evaluated that has the capability to reach victims within a time frame that is appropriate for the permit-space hazards identified and is equipped for and proficient in performing the needed rescue services.

The rescue team or service must be informed of the hazards it may confront when called on to perform rescue at the site. It also must be provided access to all permit spaces from which rescue may be necessary so it can both develop rescue plans and practice rescue operations.

On-site rescue teams

Employees who have been designated to provide permit-space rescue and emergency services must be provided with the PPE needed to conduct rescues safely and must be trained in the use of PPE, at no cost.

The employer must train the team to perform assigned rescue duties. The rescuers also must establish proficiency as authorized permit-space entrants.

The team must be trained in basic first aid and CPR. At least one member of the rescue team must hold a current certification in first aid and CPR. Designated rescue personnel must practice making permit-space rescues at least annually.

The practice sessions must simulate rescue operations in which they remove dummies, mannequins, or actual persons from the actual permit spaces or from representative permit spaces. Representative permit spaces must, with respect to opening size, configuration, and accessibility, simulate the types of permit spaces from which rescue may be necessary.

Retrieval systems

Whenever an authorized entrant enters a permit-space, retrieval systems must be used to simplify nonentry rescues, unless the retrieval equipment would increase the overall risk of entry or would not contribute to the rescue of the entrant.

Each authorized entrant must wear a chest or full-body harness, with a retrieval line attached at the center of the entrant's back near shoulder level. The line also may be attached above the entrant's head or at another point that presents a profile small enough for the successful removal of the entrant. Wristlets may be used if the employer can demonstrate that the use of a chest or full-body harness is infeasible or creates a greater hazard.

The other end of the retrieval line must be attached to a mechanical device or fixed point outside the permit space. A mechanical device must be available to retrieve personnel from vertical-type permit spaces more than 5 feet deep.

MSDS

If an injured entrant is exposed to a substance for which an MSDS is required, the medical facility that treats the exposed worker must be provided with the MSDS or other similar information.

Contractors

When an employer (host) arranges to have employees of another employer (contractor) perform work that involves permit-space entry, the host employer has specific responsibilities. These include

- informing the contractor that the workplace contains permit spaces and that permit-space entry is contingent on compliance with a permit-space program that meets the standard's requirements
- informing the contractor of the elements, including the hazards identified and the host employer's experience with the space, that make the space in question a permit space
- ensuring that the contractor knows of any precautions or procedures that the host employer has created for the protection of employees in or near permit spaces where contractor personnel will be working

- coordinating entry operations with the contractor, when both host employer personnel and contractor personnel will be working in or near permit spaces

- debriefing the contractor at the conclusion of the entry operations regarding which permit-space program was followed and regarding any hazards confronted or created in permit spaces during entry operations

In addition to complying with the permit-space requirements that apply to all employers, each contractor who is retained to perform permit-space-entry operations must

- obtain any available information regarding permit-space hazards and entry operations from the host employer

- coordinate entry operations with the host employer when both host-employer personnel and contractor personnel will be working in or near permit spaces

- inform the host employer of the permit-space program that the contractor will follow and of any hazards confronted or created in permit spaces, either through a debriefing or during the entry operations

Alternative protection

The standard allows alternative protection procedures for entry of permit spaces where the only hazard is atmospheric and ventilation alone can control the hazard. If employers use alternative protection procedures for confined-space entry, these requirements apply:

- Any condition that makes it unsafe to remove an entrance cover must be eliminated before the cover is removed.

- When entrance covers are removed, the opening must be properly guarded to protect employees from falling through and to protect those in the space from falling objects.

- Before any employee enters the space, the internal atmosphere must be tested with a calibrated direct-reading instrument for the following conditions in the order given: oxygen content, flammable gases and vapors, and potential toxic air contaminants.

- There may be no hazardous atmosphere within the space whenever any employee is inside the space.

- Continuous forced air ventilation must be used to eliminate any hazardous atmosphere.

- The atmosphere within the space must be periodically tested as necessary to ensure that the continuous forced air ventilation is preventing the accumulation of a hazardous atmosphere.

- The employer must verify that the space is safe for entry and that requirements have been met through a written certification that contains the date, location of the space, and signature of the person who provides the certification. The certification must be made before entry and be made available to each employee who enters the space.

- Employees must exit immediately if a hazardous atmosphere is detected during entry, and the space must be evaluated to determine how the hazardous atmosphere developed.

When there are changes in the use or configuration of a nonpermit confined space that might increase the hazards to entrants, the employer must reevaluate that space and, if necessary, reclassify it as a permit-required confined space.

Construction/renovation (1926)

at a glance

The construction standard presents a wide set of requirements to protect employees from injuries at construction or renovation sites.

Ensuring the safety and health of laboratory workers, visitors, and construction workers during facility construction or renovation projects involves multiple operations and crews, changing hazards, and short-term work sites. OSHA requires the creation of job-site safety and health programs by all employers involved in construction or renovation projects, including general contractors and all subcontractors. Worker-protection requirements fall under OSHA's construction-industry standards (29 CFR 1926) and general industry standards (29 CFR 1910).

OSHA standards applicable to the construction industry (29 CFR 1926) include provisions for inspections, citations, and proposed penalties; recordkeeping and reporting; PPE and life-saving equipment; fire prevention and protection; signs, signals, and barricades; handling toxic and hazardous substances; and other occupational safety and health issues.

It is the responsibility of the employer to initiate and maintain the job-site safety and health program and to designate competent persons where necessary to assist in carrying it out. The competent person usually will be designated by the subcontractor whose work is covered by a standard that requires a competent person. The general contractor does not need to provide a competent person as long as it can ensure that a competent person has been appointed.

OSHA has included all relevant mandatory standards in its construction resource manual, *Safety and Health Standards for the Construction Industry* (OSHA 3149, 1996).

Subcontractor responsibilities

Competent persons designated by subcontractors must be capable of identifying both existing and predictable hazards and must have the authority to prevent or correct the conditions. They also must have authority to perform all required activities and all aspects of the job-site program, including

- prohibiting the use of any tool, machinery, material, or equipment that is not in compliance with safety standards
- identifying and locking the controls or removing from the job site all tools, machines, materials, and equipment that do not comply with safety standards
- allowing only employees qualified by training or experience to operate equipment and machinery
- instructing employees in the recognition and avoidance of unsafe conditions
- instructing employees in the safety and health regulations applicable to their work

Multi-employer work sites

Employee exposure to hazards on a multi-employer work site may result in citations from OSHA to each exposing employer or to the employer in the best position to either correct the hazard or ensure its correction.

On multi-employer work sites (in all industry sectors), more than one employer may be citable for a hazardous condition that violates an OSHA standard. A two-step process must be followed in determining whether more than one employer is to be cited. In most cases, the general contractor hired by a laboratory, rather than the laboratory itself, is responsible for preventing and correcting hazards.

Step one

The first step is to determine whether the employer is a creating, exposing, correcting, or controlling employer, and whether the employer has multiple roles. Once the role of the employer is determined, go to Step two to determine whether a citation is appropriate. (Only exposing employers can be cited for general-duty-clause violations.)

Step two

If the employer falls into one of these roles, it has obligations under OSHA requirements. Step two determines whether the employer's actions were sufficient to meet those obligations. Tables 1, 2, 3, and 4 present scenarios to consider.

Table 1 **Creating employer**

Condition	The creating employer actually creates the hazard. A creating employer that creates violative conditions is citable, even if the only employees exposed are those of other employers at the site.
Scenario	Employer Host operates a factory and contracts with Company S to service machinery. Host fails to cover drums of a chemical despite S's repeated requests to do so. This results in airborne levels of the chemical that exceed the PEL.
Who is the creating employer?	Host is a creating employer because it caused employees of S to be exposed to the air contaminant above the PEL.
Is the employer citable?	Host failed to carry out measures to prevent the accumulation of the air contaminant. It could have met its OSHA obligation by enabling the simple engineering control of covering the drums. Having failed to use a feasible engineering control to meet the PEL, Host is citable for the hazard.

Table 2 — Exposing employer

Condition	The exposing employer's own employees are exposed to the hazard. If the exposing employer created the violation, it is citable as a creating employer. If the violation was created by another employer, the exposing employer is citable if it • knew of the condition or failed to exercise reasonable diligence to discover the condition • failed to take steps to protect its employees If the exposing employer has authority to correct the hazard, it must do so. If the employer lacks that authority, it is citable if it fails to do each of the following: • Ask the creating and/or controlling employer to correct the hazard • Inform its employees of the hazard • Take reasonable alternative protective measures – In extreme circumstances, the exposing employer is citable for failing to remove its employees from the job to avoid the hazard
Scenario	Employer Sub S is responsible for inspecting and cleaning a work area in Plant P around a large, permanent hole at the end of each day. An OSHA standard requires guardrails. There are no guardrails around the hole, and Sub S employees do not use personal fall protection, although it would be feasible to do so. Sub S has no authority to install guardrails. However, it did ask Employer P, which operates the plant, to install them. P refused. Sub S is an exposing employer because its employees are exposed to the fall hazard.
Who is the exposing employer?	Although Sub S has no authority to install guardrails, it is required to comply with OSHA requirements. It must take steps to protect its employees and ask the employer that controls the hazard to correct it. Sub S asked for guardrails, but the hazard was not corrected.
Is the employer citable?	Sub S was responsible for taking reasonable alternative protective steps, such as providing personal fall protection. Because that was not done, Sub S is citable for the violation.

Table 3

Correcting employer

Condition	The correcting employer is responsible for safety and health conditions on the work site and has the authority to ensure that the hazardous condition is corrected. The correcting employer must exercise reasonable care in preventing and discovering violations and must meet its obligations of correcting the hazard.
Scenario	Employer C, a carpentry contractor, is hired to erect and maintain guardrails throughout a large, 15-story project. C inspects all floors every morning and afternoon. It also inspects areas where material is delivered. Other subcontractors are required to report damaged or missing guardrails to the general contractor, who forwards those reports to C. C makes immediate repairs. Shortly after an afternoon inspection of Floor 6, workers accidentally damage a guardrail in one area. No one notifies C. An OSHA inspection occurs the next day, prior to the morning inspection of Floor 6. None of C's employees is exposed to the hazard, but other employees are.
Who is the correcting employer?	C is a correcting employer since it is responsible for erecting and maintaining fall protection equipment.
Is the employer citable?	The steps C carried out to discover and correct damaged guardrails were reasonable in light of the amount of activity and size of the project. It exercised reasonable care to prevent and discover violations. C is not citable for the damaged guardrail because it could not reasonably have known of the violation.

Table 4

Controlling employer

Condition	The controlling employer has the power to correct violations or require others to correct them. A controlling employer must exercise reasonable care to prevent and detect violations.
Scenario	Employer GH contracts with Employer S to do sandblasting at GH's plant. Some of the work is regularly scheduled maintenance and general industry work; other parts of the project are considered construction. Respiratory protection is required. Further, the contract explicitly requires S to comply with safety and health requirements. Under the contract, GH has the right to take various actions against S for failing to meet contract requirements, including the right to have noncompliance corrected by using other workers and back-charging for that work. S is one of two employers under contract with GH at the work site, where a total of five employees work. All work is done within an existing building. The number and types of hazards involved in S's work do not significantly change as the work progresses. Further, GH has worked with S over the course of several years. S provides periodic and other safety and health training and uses a graduated system of enforcement of safety and health rules. S has consistently had a high level of compliance at its previous jobs and at this site. GH monitors S using a combination of weekly inspections, telephone discussions, and a weekly review of S's own inspection reports. GH has a system of graduated enforcement that it has applied to S for the few safety and health violations that have been committed by S in the past few years. Further, due to respirator equipment problems, S violates respiratory protection requirements two days before GH's next scheduled inspection of S. The next day there is an OSHA inspection. There is no notation of the equipment problems in S's inspection reports to GH, and S made no mention of it in its telephone discussions.

Table 4: Controlling employer (cont.)

Who is the controlling employer?	GH is a controlling employer because it has general supervisory authority over the work site, including contractual authority to correct safety and health violations.
Is the employer citable?	GH has taken reasonable steps to try to make sure that S meets safety and health requirements. Its inspection frequency is appropriate in light of the low number of workers at the site, lack of significant changes in the nature of the work and types of hazards involved, GH's knowledge of S's history of compliance, and its effective safety and health efforts on this job. GH has exercised reasonable care and is not citable for this condition.

Hazard communication

Under OSHA's hazard-communication standard (29 CFR 1910.1200); at multi-employer work sites, employers who produce, use, or store hazardous chemicals at a workplace in such a way that the employees of other employers (e.g., employees of a construction contractor who work on-site) may be exposed must additionally ensure that the hazard communication programs developed include the following:

- The methods the employer will use to provide the other employers with on-site access to an MSDS for each hazardous chemical to which their employees may be exposed while working

- The methods the employer will use to inform the other employers of any precautionary measures that need to be taken to protect employees during the workplace's normal operating conditions and in foreseeable emergencies

- The methods the employer will use to inform the other employers of the labeling system used in the workplace

The employer may rely on an existing hazard-communication program to comply with these requirements, provided that it meets criteria of the hazard-communication standard. The written program must be available, upon request, to employees, their designated representatives, or OSHA.

Where employees must travel between workplaces during a workshift (e.g., their work is carried out at more than one geographical location), the written hazard-communication program may be kept at the primary workplace facility.

Respiratory protection

OSHA requires employers, including those at multi-employer work-sites, to use engineering controls to prevent occupational diseases caused by breathing air contaminated with harmful dusts, fumes, mists, gases, sprays, and vapors. Where effective engineering controls are not feasible or while they are being installed, respirators should be used in accordance with requirements of OSHA's respiratory-protection standard (29 CFR 1910.134).

Training requirements

OSHA requires employers to instruct each employee in the recognition and avoidance of unsafe conditions and the regulations applicable to the work environment to control or eliminate any hazards or other exposure to illness or injury.

The employer should permit only employees qualified by training or experience to operate equipment and machinery.

All employers with employees exposed to hazardous chemicals are required to train those employees in accordance with the hazard-communication standard. Employees required to handle or use poisons, caustics, and other harmful substances must be instructed in safe handling and use and be made aware of the potential hazards, personal hygiene, and personal protective measures required.

Employees required to handle or use flammable liquids, gases, or toxic materials must be instructed in the safe handling and use of these materials and be made aware of specific requirements.

All employees required to enter confined or enclosed spaces must be instructed as to the nature of the hazards involved, the necessary precautions to be taken, and the use of protective and emergency equipment required. The employer must comply with any specific regulations that apply to work in dangerous or potentially dangerous areas.

Inspection procedures

During a construction inspection, a compliance safety and health officer must complete an evaluation of the safety and health program to determine whether an effective program is being maintained. The degree of knowledge employees have about potential site-specific safety and health hazards is reviewed in the evaluation. The compliance safety and health officer then discusses the findings with the employer. Any deficiencies in the program—such as lack of management policy or safety and health rules, inadequate assignment of responsibility, or poor employee awareness/participation—also are discussed at that time.

Violations of requirements for instruction, first aid, recordkeeping, and identification and control of hazards may be cited as set forth in the construction standard. If a citation is necessary for violation of safety and health provisions or safety training and education, it can be issued even if other alleged violations of the standard are not documented.

Asbestos hazards

Asbestos is defined under both the general industry and the construction standards as including chrysotile, amosite, crocidolite, tremolite asbestos, anthophyllite asbestos, actinolite asbestos, and any of these minerals that have been chemically treated or altered. The definition does not include nonasbestiform varieties of the minerals tremolite, anthophyllite, and actinolite, which may be covered under OSHA's air-contaminants standard (29 CFR 1910.1000) as particulates not otherwise regulated.

The construction standard (29 CFR 1926.1101) covers asbestos hazards related to demolition, renovation, or maintenance, regardless of the employer's primary business. Such work is divided into classes (Class I, II, III, and IV) that correspond to the level of exposure hazard. The extent of controls required depends on the classification of the work. Generally, however, employers must

- appoint a competent person to supervise asbestos-related work
- conduct initial exposure monitoring at the start of each asbestos job
- establish regulated areas for asbestos jobs, with posted warnings and restricted access
- use wet methods to control fiber dispersion during asbestos work and HEPA-filter vacuums to clean up asbestos dust and debris, and ensure prompt disposal of asbestos-containing material

Lead hazards

The OSHA construction-industry lead standard (29 CFR 1926.62) applies to all construction work in which an employee could be exposed to lead, including alteration and repair involving painting and decorating. It includes but is not limited to the following:

- Demolition or salvage of structures where lead or materials that contain lead are present
- Removal or encapsulation of materials containing lead
- New construction, alteration, repair, or renovation of structures, substrates, or portions thereof that contain lead or materials that contain lead

- Installation of products containing lead
- Lead contamination and emergency cleanup
- Transportation, disposal, storage, or containment of lead or materials that contain lead on the site or location at which construction activities are performed
- Maintenance operations associated with construction activities

Employers must create engineering and work-practice controls, including administrative controls, to reduce and maintain employee exposure to lead at or below the PEL, to the extent that such controls are feasible. When these controls are not sufficient to reduce exposure to below the PEL, the employer must use them fully and supplement them with respiratory protection.

When ventilation is used to control lead exposure, the employer must evaluate the mechanical performance of the system as necessary to maintain its effectiveness. If administrative controls are used as a means of reducing exposure, the employer must establish a job rotation schedule that includes the name or identification number of each affected employee, duration and exposure levels at each job or work station, and any other information useful in assessing the reliability of administrative controls.

Methylene chloride exposure

OSHA's methylene chloride standard applies to employers in general industry (29 CFR 1910.1052) and in the construction industry (29 CFR 1926.1152). The standard includes requirements for exposure control, PPE, employee exposure monitoring, employee training, medical surveillance, hazard communication, and recordkeeping.

Methylene chloride is a solvent with a chloroform-like odor used for paint removal, metal degreasing, and certain pharmaceutical and aerosol products. Exposure often occurs when workers strip paint or other coatings, apply foam, paint with epoxy paint, clean equipment with solvents, and spray adhesives.

Worker exposures to methylene chloride occur mainly through breathing its vapors, but the substance also can pass through workers' skin if it gets on their bodies or clothes. Short-term exposure to high levels of methylene chloride can cause irritation of the skin, eyes, and respiratory system, as well as dizziness and headaches.

Exposure limits

OSHA has established a PEL for methylene chloride of 25 ppm as an eight-hour TWA; a STEL of 125 ppm during a sampling period of 15 minutes; and an action level of 12.5 ppm calculated as an eight-hour TWA. Employee exposure at or above the action level indicates that the employer must initiate compliance activities such as monitoring and medical surveillance.

Where employee exposure to airborne concentrations of methylene chloride exceeds or can be reasonably expected to exceed either the eight-hour PEL or 15-minute STEL, regulated areas should be established with access limited to authorized personnel.

Conveniently located washing facilities and emergency eyewash facilities must be provided in areas where exposure to methylene chloride may occur. Contaminated clothing should be removed immediately, and affected areas of the body should be washed thoroughly with soap and water.

Substitutes

To reduce worker exposures, OSHA recommends the use of paint strippers, adhesives, solvents, foams, and paints that do not contain methylene chloride.

Emergency eyewash facilities

OSHA's medical and first-aid standard requirement (29 CFR 1910.151) for eyewash and body-drench facilities is applicable to construction activities.

Specifically, at construction sites, eyewash and body-drench equipment should be provided within 100 feet of work stations at locations where hazardous chemicals are handled by employees. When locating eyewash stations, attention should be paid to the physical layout of the work area and obstructions such as machinery and equipment. The employee, who may be partly blinded by chemicals in the eyes, must be able to reach and use eyewash and/or body-drench facilities within 10 seconds. Nozzles on eyewash units should be protected with airtight but easily removable covers to prevent airborne contamination and to prevent freezing of water in cold weather.

Electrical safety (1910, subpart S)

at a glance

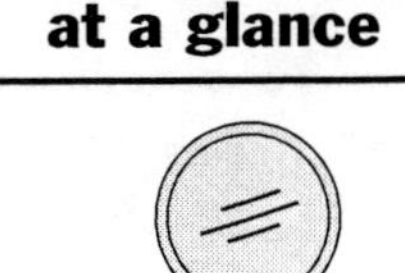

The electrical safety standard protects employees from electric shock and other related injuries.

Electrical safety

Electrical equipment shall be free from recognized hazards that are likely to cause death or serious physical harm to employees (29 CFR 1910.303[b][1]).

All electrical equipment, including building electrical-system components and tools that use electrical power, must be tested and accepted by an OSHA-recognized testing laboratory (29 CFR 1910.303[b][2]).

Flexible cords and cables (extension cords)

Flexible cords and cables shall be protected from accidental damage (29 CFR 1910.305[a][2][iii][G]).

Unless specifically permitted, flexible cords and cables may not be used

- as substitutes for the fixed wiring of a structure
- where attached to building surfaces
- where concealed
- where run through holes in walls, ceilings, or floors
- where run through doorways, windows, or similar openings.

Flexible cords shall be connected to devices and fittings so that strain relief is provided that will prevent pull from being directly transmitted to joints or terminal screws (29 CFR 1910.305[g][2][iii]).

Grounding/grounded

For a grounded system, a grounding electrode conductor shall be used to connect both the equipment-grounding conductor and the grounded circuit conductor to the grounding electrode. Both the equipment-grounding conductor and the grounding electrode conductor shall be connected to the grounded circuit conductor on the supply side of the service disconnecting means or on the supply side of the system disconnecting means (or overcurrent devices, if the system is separately derived) (29 CFR 1910.304[f][3][i]).

For an ungrounded service-supplied system, the equipment-grounding conductor must be connected to the grounding electrode conductor at the service equipment (29 CFR 1910.304[f][3][ii]).

The path to ground from circuits, equipment, and enclosures must be permanent and continuous (29 CFR 1910.304[f][4]).

Guarding

Electrical equipment shall be free from recognized hazards that are likely to cause death or serious physical harm to employees (29 CFR 1910.303[b][1]).

Identification

Each disconnecting means shall be legibly marked to indicate its purpose, unless it is located and arranged so the purpose is evident (29 CFR 1910.303[f]).

Listing and labeling

Listed or labeled equipment shall be used or installed in accordance with any instructions included in the listing or labeling (29 CFR 1910.303[b][2]).

Openings

Unused openings in cabinets, boxes, and fittings shall be effectively closed (29 CFR 1910.305[b][1]).

Safety-related work practices

Safety-related work practices shall be employed to prevent electric shock or other injuries that result from either direct or indirect electrical contacts when work is performed near or on equipment or circuits that are or may be energized (29 CFR 1910.333[a]).

Electrical safety-related work practices cover both qualified persons (those who have training in avoiding the electrical hazards of working on or near exposed energized parts) and unqualified persons (those with little or no such training) (29 CFR 1910.331[a]). There must be written lockout and/or tagout procedures (this may be a copy of 1910.333[b][2]) (29 CFR 1910.333[b][2][i]).

Overhead power lines must be deenergized and grounded by the owner or operator of the lines, or other protective measures must be provided before work is started. Protective measures, such as guarding or insulating the lines, must be designed to prevent employees from contacting the lines (29 CFR 1910.333[c][3]).

Unqualified employees and mechanical equipment must be at least 10 feet away from overhead power lines. If the voltage exceeds 50,000 volts, the clearance distance should be increased four inches for each additional 10,000 volts (29 CFR 1910.333[c][3][i] and [iii]).

OSHA requires portable ladders to have nonconductive side rails if used by employees who would be working where they might contact exposed energized circuit parts (29 CFR 1910.333[c][7]).

Splices

Conductors must be spliced or joined with devices identified for such use or by brazing, welding, or soldering with a fusible alloy or metal. All splices, joints, and free ends of conductors must be covered with an insulation equivalent to that of the conductor or with an insulating device suitable for the purpose (29 CFR 1910.303[c]).

Emergency plans (1910.38)

at a glance

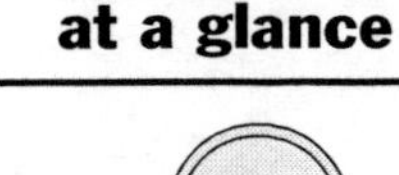

The emergency plans standard sets requirements for having emergency-action plans in place.

Wherever any given OSHA standard requires one, the employer will create an emergency plan to ensure employee safety. The standard requires a written plan that you should make available in facilities with 11 or more employees. In facilities with 10 or fewer employees, an employer may communicate the plan orally to employees.

Emergency action plans should address emergencies that the employer may reasonably expect in the workplace. Examples are fire, toxic chemical releases, hurricanes, tornadoes, blizzards, floods, bombings, and bioterror acts.

Plan requirements

The emergency plan must include, at a minimum, the following elements:

- Emergency escape procedures and escape routes
- Procedures for employees who remain to perform or shut down critical office operations
- Procedures to account for all employees after the completion of an emergency evacuation
- Rescue and medical duties for those employees responsible for performing them
- The procedures for and preferred means of reporting fires and other emergencies
- The names or regular job titles of persons or departments you need to contact for further information or explanation of duties under the plan

Alarm system

An employer must have and maintain an employee alarm system. The employee alarm system must use a distinctive signal for each purpose and comply with the requirements in the OSHA employee alarm systems standard 1910.165.

For those employers with 10 or fewer employees, direct voice communication is an acceptable procedure for sounding an alarm, provided that all employees can hear the alarm.

Review

An employer must review the emergency action plan with each employee covered by the plan on the following occasions:

- Upon creation of the plan
- With an employee's initial job assignment
- When the employee's responsibilities under the plan change
- When the plan changes

Ensure that emergency plans reasonably cover all employees. For example, a single emergency plan for the primary worksite may not be adequate for auxiliary sites or for employees working off-site.

Emergency response/HAZWOPER (1910.120)

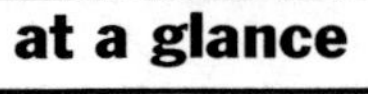

at a glance

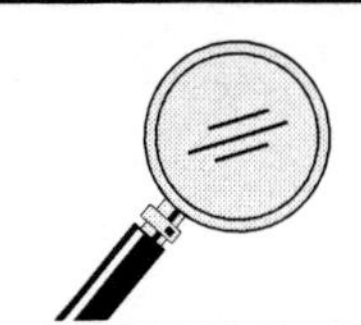

The emergency response/HAZWOPER standard sets requirements for workers who must respond to hazardous-substance spills.

OSHA's HAZWOPER rule (29 CFR 1910.120) requires that employers develop a written emergency-response plan to handle possible emergencies before performing hazardous-waste operations. The plan must include various provisions, depending on what type of site or incident is involved. Different provisions may apply for emergency response at the following:

- Uncontrolled hazardous-waste sites
- RCRA-permitted hazardous-waste treatment, storage, and disposal facilities
- Hazardous-substance releases

Emergency response to hazardous-substance releases

Under the standard (29 CFR 1910.120[q]), employers that engage in emergency-response operations for release of, or substantial threats of release of, hazardous substances without regard to the location of the hazard must have a plan that includes the following:

- Preemergency planning and coordination with outside parties
- Safe distances and places of refuge
- Site security and control
- Evacuation routes and procedures
- Decontamination
- Emergency medical treatment and first aid
- Emergency alerting and response procedures
- Critique of response and follow-up
- PPE and emergency equipment

The HAZWOPER standard requires laboratories to plan for external emergencies if they expect to use their employees to handle an emergency that involves hazardous substances.

Employees who participate, or are expected to participate, in an emergency response to hazardous-substance releases must be given training, the extent of which depends on their involvement and responsibilities. Laboratories in hospitals must have emergency-response plans that meet JCAHO guidelines.

According to OSHA, the plans must include provisions for the following:

- Training employees
- Documenting training
- Performing emergency drills
- Defining personnel roles
- Responding to emergencies
- Selecting PPE (including respirators)
- Decontaminating patients
- Avoiding cross-contamination

Inspection procedures

According to OSHA-inspection procedures for emergency response to hazardous-substance releases, one of the most important aspects of HAZWOPER is planning for emergencies through the development of an emergency-response plan or an emergency action plan (OSHA Instruction CPL 2-2.59A).

During an inspection of a facility's emergency-response program, OSHA inspectors must review the following elements:

- Emergency-response plan
- Procedures for handling emergencies

- Training requirements
- Medical-surveillance provisions
- PPE program

The compliance officer also may conduct employee interviews to measure knowledge of the facility's emergency-response procedures.

When reviewing the emergency-response plan, the compliance officer must evaluate the employer's ability to contain, control, and clean up hazardous substances if an emergency occurs. If a facility does not have an emergency-response plan or an emergency action plan, the employer must prove that the chemicals and quantities of them used in the facility will not develop into an emergency incident if released in a reasonably predictable worst-case scenario. If there is a potential for an emergency, the employer must plan for it, and if there is no potential, then the employer does not fall within the scope of HAZWOPER.

Incidental releases

OSHA also provides guidance on the types of releases that require an emergency response. Although HAZWOPER may not apply, incidental chemical releases still are covered by the OSHA hazard-communication standard, 29 CFR 1910.1200. Inspectors are instructed by OSHA to check what, if any, written procedures exist in the employer's written hazard-communication program for handling incidental releases.

Laboratory facilities may be covered under HAZWOPER in at least three scenarios:

- When facilities have an internal release of a hazardous substance that requires an emergency response
- When facilities respond as an integral unit in a community-wide emergency response to a release of a hazardous substance
- If a facility is an RCRA-permitted hazardous-waste treatment, storage, and disposal facility

Definition of hazardous substance

For the purposes of the HAZWOPER standard, OSHA expanded on the Superfund definition of "hazardous substance." In addition to CERCLA-listed hazardous substances, DOT-regulated hazardous materials (e.g., chemicals or radioactive materials), and RCRA- and DOT-regulated hazardous wastes, OSHA includes in its definition of hazardous substance "any biological agent and other disease-causing agent which after release into the environment and upon exposure, ingestion, inhalation, or assimilation into any person, either directly from the environment or indirectly by ingestion through food chains, will be or may reasonably be anticipated to cause death, disease, behavioral abnormalities, cancer, genetic mutation, physiological malfunctions—including malfunctions in reproduction—or physical deformations in such persons or their offspring."

The agency also includes petroleum products and gases as hazardous-waste materials covered under the standard.

Response to an internal spill

Certain HAZWOPER requirements about employees who may have to respond to a spill or release of hazardous substances within the facility boundaries apply to laboratory facilities. Such releases may be covered by the emergency response to hazardous-substance release provisions of the standard (29 CFR 1910.120[q]). Associated training requirements also apply.

To determine how much training an in-house employee must receive, the employer must consider the degree of hazard involved using worst-case scenarios. The key factor in this determination is the actual or estimated hazard exposure or degree of danger to employees and other persons. Another consideration is whether the facility is managing the spill or contracting for hazardous substance spill services. With a contract for services, training may be minimal—initiating a spill response call and securing the area, for example.

Incidental release

An incidental release does not pose an imminent health or safety hazard that requires immediate cleanup to prevent death or serious injury, and housekeeping staff can safely clean it up without danger to themselves. Cleanups of such releases are not considered emergency responses and therefore are not covered under the HAZWOPER training requirements. Other training requirements, such as those imposed under the OSHA Hazard Communication Standard, would apply.

Emergency response

If the employer determines that the potential exists for an emergency to develop, then employees must receive, as a minimum, first-responder awareness-level training. Several different levels of training are required for emergency responders, depending on their responsibilities and the hazards they face.

The training must be designed to enable workers to distinguish a nonemergency incidental release from a release that is beyond their ability to handle without danger to themselves. The training also must instruct employees about how to initiate emergency procedures. Because medical and infectious wastes are included in the HAZWOPER definition of hazardous substances, laboratory facilities must include such wastes in their effort to comply with the standard's training requirements.

All employees, regardless of title, must be trained to perform their assigned job duties in a safe and healthful manner. Staff who are expected to handle cleanup of medical waste and infectious materials in laboratory settings in nonemergency situations must be trained in accordance with OSHA's bloodborne-pathogens standard. Cleanup of other hazardous substances, such as mercury from a broken thermometer, would necessitate training under the OSHA Hazard Communication Standard.

Facility emergency-response plan

Laboratory facilities may be required to develop emergency-response plans under HAZWOPER. Under the standard, the plan must designate personnel roles, a "senior official," and lines of authority. Also, the plan may include evacuation procedures for employees and patients and may be a part of the facility's internal disaster plan.

If the facility elects to designate an in-house staff member as the incident commander during an emergency, this person must meet the HAZWOPER training requirements for such individuals. The incident commander also must be able to carry out the standard's procedures for handling an emergency response. An incident commander is not required to be on-site at all times, but he or she would have to be on call 24 hours a day. The facility's emergency-response plan must identify the most senior official who will be in charge until the designated incident commander arrives.

The facility also may enlist outside assistance, such as the fire department, during an on-site emergency spill. OSHA advises that the assistance of outside emergency responders be coordinated in the facility's emergency-response plan prior to an emergency-response incident.

Response to ethylene oxide (EtO) releases

Because of the hazards that EtO presents, most leaks would require an emergency response, according to OSHA. Any laboratory facility worker who is expected to handle releases of EtO should receive training that enables the worker to handle worst-case scenarios safely. This likely would entail compliance with HAZWOPER training requirements.

Compliance with OSHA's Ethylene Oxide Standard also is required (29 CFR 1910.1047). That standard imposes requirements for medical surveillance, handling procedures, and training that are specific to the hazards of the substance. The worker need only be trained to meet HAZWOPER training requirements, which meet and go beyond those under the EtO standard.

Facility role in community emergency response

Laboratory workers who deal with external emergencies may be exposed to chemical, biological, physical, or radioactive hazards. Protecting workers who respond to emergencies that involve hazardous substances is critical. Laboratories that provide emergency-response services must be prepared to carry out their missions without jeopardizing the safety and health of their workers.

Of special concern are situations in which contaminated patients arrive at the hospital for triage or definitive treatment following a major incident. OSHA, in January 2005, issued *Best Practices for Hospital-Based First Receivers of Victims from Mass Casualty Incidents Involving the Release of Hazardous Substances,* which consolidates the agency's related requirements for training first receivers and instructs hospitals on decontaminating patients and selecting PPE. The guidelines are not new, nor are they mandatory; however, OSHA inspectors may monitor whether hospitals and laboratories within hospitals use these best practices. The Best Practices document is available on the OSHA Web site at *www.osha.gov/dts/osta/bestpractices/firstreceivers_hospital.html.*

RCRA-permitted facilities

If a laboratory is permitted under RCRA as a hazardous-waste treatment, storage, and disposal facility, the employees who work at the facility must be trained according to HAZWOPER requirements under 29 CFR 1910.120(p). This would apply, for example, to a laboratory that had a medical-waste incinerator that was permitted under RCRA to burn hazardous waste as well. The training requirements apply only to employees who work at the TSD facility itself, not to employees working anywhere at the healthcare facility.

Training requirements

Emergency response

Training must be based on the duties and functions of the responder in an emergency-response organization. The skill and knowledge levels required for all new responders must be conveyed through training before they are permitted to take part in an actual emergency operation. There are five levels of emergency responders, and each level has different training requirements.

First-responder awareness level

First responders at the awareness level are individuals likely to witness or discover a hazardous-substance release and initiate emergency response by notifying the proper authorities of the release. First responders at the awareness level must be trained to understand what hazardous substances are and the risks associated with them in an incident, understand potential outcomes of emergencies created by hazardous substances, recognize the presence of hazardous substances in an emergency and identify the substances, understand the role of the first-responder awareness individual in the employer's emergency-response plan, realize when additional resources are needed, and make appropriate notifications to the communication center.

First-responder operations level

First responders at the operations level are trained to respond defensively without actually trying to stop the release. Their function is to contain the release from a safe distance, keep it from spreading, and prevent exposures. First responders must demonstrate competency; be certified in requirements for the awareness level; be trained to know basic hazard and risk-assessment techniques; use and select proper PPE; perform basic control, containment, or confinement operations with available resources; implement basic decontamination procedures; and understand relevant standard operating and termination procedures.

Laboratories may either develop an in-house training course on decontamination and PPE use and on measures to prevent the spread of contamination to other portions of the facility or provide additional training in decontamination and PPE use after sending personnel to a standard first-responder operations-level course.

All laboratory employees, including ancillary personnel such as housekeeping staff, must be adequately trained to perform their assigned job duties in a safe and healthful manner. If laboratory personnel will be expected to clean up the decontamination area, they must be trained in accordance with 29 CFR 1910.120(q)(11) and have access to MSDSs for those chemicals that may be used to decontaminate the equipment and area. Coordination with community resources for cleanup assistance should be included in the contingency plan.

Employee health services

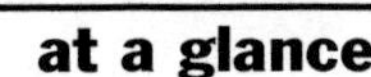

at a glance

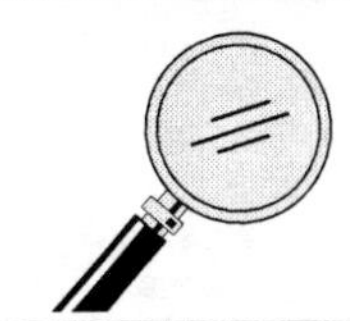

In many cases, the employee health services (EHS) provide medical services that OSHA requires under other standards.

Protecting workers from the multitude of occupational hazards that may be present in the laboratory setting is a challenge for many employers.

The major objectives of an EHS are to provide a safe and healthful work environment, as required by OSHA, and to provide employees with the services they need to maintain optimum health while working in the laboratory. To accomplish these objectives, employee laboratory professionals need to be knowledgeable about job areas, processes, job descriptions, and potential exposures to hazardous substances in their facilities. In many cases, the EHS provides medical services that are required under workplace standards issued by OSHA.

The EHS usually is not considered to be a replacement for private medical care. Employers may want to emphasize to employees that despite the provision of certain medical services, their healthcare ultimately remains their own responsibility.

Structure and services

For an EHS to function properly, laboratory administration must invest in it appropriate responsibility, authority, and funding to carry out its duties.

In most cases, the EHS performs an array of functions. One of the most important is the tracking of employee illnesses and injuries. These data, which must be reported to OSHA, are useful for improving the laboratory's overall safety performance because they help to pinpoint areas where effort should be focused on prevention rather than treatment. Medical monitoring required under specific federal workplace-safety standards also may be administered through the EHS.

Employee health programs should provide at least the following:

- Preplacement physical exams, including a complete medical history
- Periodic health-appraisal examinations
- Health and safety education
- Immunizations
- Care for illness and injury at work
- Health counseling
- Environmental control and surveillance
- Health and safety records system
- Coordination with other departments and services, such as infection control and radiation safety

Infection-control guidelines

If the laboratory is part of a hospital or other larger facility, the activities of the personnel health service should be coordinated with infection-control and other departmental personnel. This coordination among departments will help ensure adequate surveillance of infections in personnel and provision of preventive services. Also, such coordination will help to ensure that investigations of exposures and outbreaks are conducted efficiently and preventive measures are implemented promptly.

The following infection-control elements are necessary in an employee health program:

- Medical evaluations

- Health and safety education

- Immunization programs

- Management of job-related illnesses and exposures to infectious diseases, including policies for work restrictions for infected or exposed personnel

- Counseling services for personnel on infection risks related to employment or special conditions

- Maintenance and confidentiality of personnel health records

OSHA medical surveillance requirements

One of the major responsibilities of the EHS is to carry out medical surveillance and provide appropriate medical care to employees exposed to infectious agents and hazardous substances.

OSHA has promulgated standards that address specific workplace hazards (e.g., bloodborne pathogens, ethylene oxide, formaldehyde, asbestos, and air contaminants). The standards require employers to take specific steps, including implementation of engineering and work practice controls, to protect workers. EHS responsibilities may include initial and periodic medical exams and postexposure follow-up testing and medical treatment. Postexposure psychological counseling also may be required, such as under the bloodborne-pathogens standard. Certain medical records must be kept for each employee who is exposed and treated.

Safety managers should be reminded to forward any air-sampling results that show that employees may have been exposed to higher-than-permitted levels of hazardous substances. This will enable the EHS to identify and monitor potentially exposed workers as required by OSHA.

On-site healthcare

Many healthcare organizations offer comprehensive on-site healthcare services to employees and their dependents. Others have a policy to provide care only for occupationally related illness or injury, and to refer other medical problems to employees' personal physicians. In those cases, the EHS should have procedures in place for contacting and communicating with the private physician and ensuring continuity of care for the employee.

Whatever type of care the EHS provides, a specific site within the laboratory facility should be made available for workers to receive those medical and other consultive services on a 24-hour basis.

Generally, it is considered preferable to treat employees through a separate EHS office with its own exam room, waiting room, and clerical staff, rather than providing care through a hospital emergency room or other department used by the general public. To encourage employees to make use of the EHS, good lighting, proper ventilation, and provision of conveniences such as restrooms and a telephone should be provided. The service also should employ a competent consulting staff.

Treatment and reporting of occupational injuries and illnesses should conform to the state workers' compensation laws and to OSHA standards.

Typically, an EHS employs at least one full-time registered nurse or a nurse-practitioner. Physician services are less consistently provided and might be offered part-time only.

Safety committees and interdepartmental policymaking

Because laboratory safety hazards are numerous and diverse, a committee that represents all laboratory services should be formed to advise the administration on the policy, direction, and requirements of the EHS or other occupational health program.

A member of the EHS should be on both the safety committee and the infection-control committee. These committees should consider in their planning the health of all workers.

Mental-health services

Most experts recommend that stress management and other types of psychological and social-counseling programs be offered, either through the EHS or through an EAP.

An EAP can help shiftworkers who face the added challenge of sleepiness on the job, a situation that can lead to loss of productivity and errors on the job.

Training and assistance in good eating habits and nutrition also are valuable to staff and, ultimately, to the quality of laboratory services.

Some employers offer mental-health services for workers with various addictive problems (e.g., tobacco, drugs, food, and alcohol), as well as for those with problems associated with HIV and the HIV epidemic.

In any case, a formal system for referral and review should be provided for workers with problems that require professional intervention that is unavailable in the facility.

Program components

Specific programs offered by an EHS vary from one facility to another. The EHS may be responsible for preplacement exams, immunizations, annual physicals, periodic monitoring, and medical recordkeeping. Wellness programs such as back-injury prevention, ergonomics, stress management, smoking cessation, and weight management also may be offered.

Preplacement exams

Preplacement medical exams are used to ensure that employees are able to safely perform their jobs without posing undue risk to others. A job-specific preplacement health evaluation is recommended for each laboratory employee and should be conducted by a qualified professional, such as an occupational-health nurse who is familiar with laboratory hazards and their effects. It should be conducted at the time of hire and whenever the employee is assigned to a new job or area. The person who conducts the exam may make a recommendation as to whether the employee can perform the job safely. However, actual hiring and job placement decisions usually are made by the personnel department and based on all appropriate medical and legal considerations.

Medical evaluations before placement can ensure that personnel are not placed in jobs that would pose undue risk of infection to them, other personnel, patients, or visitors. An important component of the placement evaluation is a health inventory. This usually includes determining immunization status and obtaining histories of any conditions that might predispose personnel to acquiring or transmitting communicable diseases. This information will simplify decisions about immunizations or postexposure management.

The preplacement exam should assess the presence of or susceptibility to communicable disease, utilizing personal interviews, medical records, and, if needed, a physical exam to determine each individual's medical history and immunization status. Of particular concern are immunization records, evidence of childhood diseases (e.g., chicken pox and measles), previous exposure to or treatment for TB, hepatitis, dermatologic conditions, chronic draining infections or open wounds, and immunodeficiency conditions. A record of the occupational history of the worker should be included in the preplacement examination.

Periodic evaluations may be done as indicated for job reassignment, ongoing programs (e.g., TB screening), or evaluation of work-related problems.

Employees generally should receive the results of their medical evaluations. In cases where infections, illnesses, or abnormalities are discovered, the employee should be informed and appropriate follow-up care recommended. Recommendations for restriction in physical activity, limitation of hazardous exposure, use of special protective measures, or other medical restrictions should be reviewed with the employee prior to job placement.

Periodic and annual physical exams

The health status of each employee should be reviewed through a periodic health assessment whenever there is a likelihood that workplace exposures or activities could have an adverse health effect. Periodic health-appraisal examinations generally are recommended for workers who are

- exposed to hazardous environments
- returning from an absence caused by illness or injury

- transferred to another department or service
- retiring

Employers may find it helpful to develop a list of job categories that require periodic evaluation, depending upon factors such as employee age, the nature and duration of the job assignment, and the degree of risk of exposure in that position. Workers exposed to certain infectious agents or potentially toxic substances such as bloodborne pathogens, TB, EtO, and formaldehyde may be entitled to receive periodic health appraisals and medical monitoring.

Postexposure follow-up

Postexposure assessment and treatment is performed after an employee has been exposed to a potentially infectious agent or other hazardous substance. Generally, the EHS should develop policies and procedures for responding to exposure incidents, such as for needlestick injuries.

Workers for whom postexposure follow-up is mandated by OSHA include those exposed to bloodborne pathogens, TB, EtO, and formaldehyde.

Immunization programs

The optimal use of vaccines can prevent transmission of some vaccine-preventable diseases and eliminate unnecessary work restriction. Mandatory immunization programs, which include both newly hired and currently employed persons, are more effective than voluntary programs in ensuring that susceptible persons are vaccinated. Also, programs in which the employer bears the cost of vaccination have had higher personnel vaccination rates than have programs without such support.

Employee-health-program immunizations may include those for diptheria, polio, tetanus, influenza, measles, mumps, rubella, and, in some cases, HBV. Elective immunizations should be considered for special situations, such as epidemics, unusual laboratory conditions, or accidental exposures (e.g., HBV needlestick incidents). A system for updating immunizations should be maintained.

Recommended vaccinations

ACIP/HICPAC guidelines strongly recommend that the following vaccinations be provided to laboratory workers, unless they show acceptable proof of vaccination or immunity:

- **Hepatitis B**—Workers whose jobs expose them to blood or OPIM (e.g., certain body fluids, sharps) should be vaccinated. Timely postexposure prophylaxis may be considered for workers whose exposure to blood is infrequent.

- **Influenza**—The influenza vaccine is recommended in the fall of each year for laboratory personnel in hospital, chronic-care, and outpatient-care settings who have contact with high-risk patients in all age groups.

- **Rubella**—Those laboratory personnel (male and female) who may be at risk of exposure to patients infected with rubella or who may have contact with pregnant patients should be vaccinated.

- **Measles**—All workers should be immunized.

- **Mumps**—Immunization is considered highly desirable for all laboratory workers.

- **Varicella**—All laboratory workers should be immune to varicella.

Environmental control and surveillance

An environmental control and surveillance program is an important part of an employee health program. It should be directed by a qualified individual or consultant who is capable of managing harmful exposures in the laboratory and who is familiar with federal and state agency regulations and requirements. A single qualified individual should be responsible for nuclear medicine and radiological activities.

Generally, the environmental engineer, industrial hygienist, and safety engineer should work cooperatively with an employee health nurse to identify potential and actual areas of risk in and around a laboratory facility. Special attention is required for maintenance areas and their supplies.

Exposure monitoring

Accidental adverse exposure to toxic chemicals can occur in various ways, such as during chemical spills, ventilation system failures, fires, and even normal working conditions. Effects of chemical exposures can range from minor skin irritations to possible carcinogenicity, teratogenicity, and mutagenicity.

EHS personnel should be especially familiar with clinical toxicology, appropriate industrial hygiene monitoring, and environmental-control methodology for all of the regulated chemical substances used in the laboratory environment.

EHS staff also should be aware of applicable federal, state, and local right-to-know laws that may require workers to be informed of the potential hazards associated with chemical substances in their workplace.

Reproductive hazards

The EHS should have a policy for counseling pregnant employees and women of childbearing age on specific hazards or potentially hazardous exposures in the laboratory. Education prior to pregnancy and cooperation with the employee's obstetrician are recommended.

Recordkeeping systems

Each worker should have a health record maintained in the health unit. The record should include all reports of the following:

- Examinations
- Treatments, medications, and immunizations
- Results of clinical tests
- Medical consultations
- Hospitalizations
- Reports of injury and illness
- Reports to and from physicians
- Exposure records

Maintenance of records on medical evaluations, immunizations, exposures, post-exposure prophylaxis, and screening tests in a retrievable (preferably computerized) database allows efficient monitoring of the health status of personnel. Such recordkeeping also helps to ensure that the organization provides consistent and appropriate services to laboratory workers.

Access to medical records

Generally, access to employee medical records should be restricted to authorized personnel only. Employees are entitled to see their own medical records under OSHA regulations. Generally, this rule provides every employee with the right of direct access to his or her own record, except in cases where the physician determines that certain information about terminal illness or psychiatric conditions could be detrimental to the employee's health. An employee's designated representative, such as a lawyer or union steward, also must be provided access upon the worker's request. Federal, state, or local laws also may restrict the disclosure of employee medical records. For example, records related to HBV or HIV status must be restricted to authorized personnel both inside and outside the facility in accordance with OSHA's bloodborne-pathogens standard. State and local regulations also may restrict disclosure of medical records. EHS personnel who maintain or provide access to employee records should fully understand their legal responsibilities and workers' rights to privacy in this area.

Ergonomics (voluntary guideline)

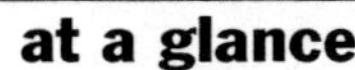

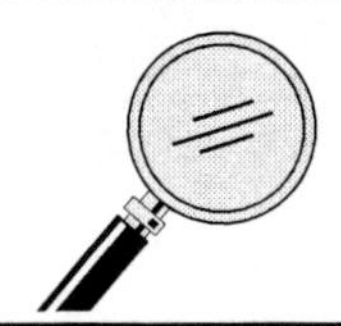

OSHA has released a few industry guidelines for ergonomics. It can also cite ergonomics deficiencies under its general duty clause.

MSDs rank high among health problems in the workplace and are a leading cause of disability among workers, according to OSHA.

Although MSDs cause few work-related deaths, they often result in human suffering, nearly 70 million visits to physicians' offices each year, loss of productivity, more than $50 billion annually in lost workdays, and an economic drain on compensation systems. In the laboratory setting, musculoskeletal stress can result from ergonomic factors such as using poorly designed furniture, lighting, and equipment, and lifting heavy materials.

The move toward automation in offices and the new technologies involved with this automation have increased the incidences of ergonomic problems such as chronic repetitive motion and static and constrained postures. Computers, video display terminals, and optical scanners are some of the high-tech tools that have generated new and pervasive sources of biomechanical stress that cause musculoskeletal problems.

OSHA's ergonomics plan is not a regulation or standard; it does not force industries to comply with its guidelines. OSHA's general duty clause, however, still imposes on employers the general obligation of furnishing workplaces that are "free from recognized hazards that are causing or are likely to cause death or serious physical harm."

Ergonomic hazards

Ergonomics includes the study of workplace equipment, environment, tasks, and personnel with the purpose of finding solutions that ease the strain on the human body. Ergonomic hazards have become an important aspect of OSHA's workplace inspections. OSHA inspectors are instructed to be alert for high incidences of ergonomic disorders listed on OSHA Form 300—Log of Work-Related Injuries and Illnesses. Inspectors also are more receptive to employee complaints of musculoskeletal problems associated with specific tasks. OSHA area offices are permitted to receive formal complaints regarding ergonomic problems. As a result, more emphasis is being placed on finding ergonomic solutions to MSDs that are likely to be encountered in workplaces.

An ergonomic study of a workplace aims to

- minimize work-related stress
- control work-related cumulative trauma illnesses and injuries
- increase job efficiency, productivity, and quality
- reduce product damage
- raise employee morale
- reduce turnover and absenteeism rates

Even without a formal ergonomics rule, OSHA can enforce MSD hazard control through its general duty clause. And you should expect that the JCAHO will include ergonomics in its survey visits. The JCAHO's EC standards include provisions that call for laboratories to keep workers safe. Laboratories must take actions to eliminate, minimize, or report safety risks.

Causes

Although the causes of occupational MSDs remain debatable, it generally is accepted that chronic exposure to physical stress tends to trigger, accelerate, or aggravate MSDs.

The sources of physical stress often can be traced to ordinary work activities that include repetitive or sustained lifting, bending, twisting, reaching, gripping, pinching, rubbing, kneeling, and squatting. When the demands of these activities repeatedly exceed the biomechanical capacity of the worker, the activities tend to induce trauma and cause MSDs.

Measures to reduce MSDs can include approaches such as conducting job analysis and redesigning the work process or tools to reduce biomechanical stress. When insufficient information regarding job processes is the problem, assumptions based on biomechanical models of physical trauma can be used.

Information available about ergonomics and related fields suggests that a majority of occupational MSDs can be eliminated if feasible ergonomic solutions are put into practice.

Job analysis

Job analysis data can help identify and assess the need for an ergonomics program in a facility. Methods for collecting this information include

- general observations
- questionnaires/interviews with employees
- videotape analysis
- photographs
- drawings or sketches

High concentrations of cumulative trauma injuries and illnesses and hazardous operations in a facility also can be identified by studying the following:

- Medical and insurance records
- Injury and illnesses analyses
- OSHA 300 Log of Work-Related Injuries and Illnesses
- Worker complaints and suggestions

Specific job hazard analysis or job safety analysis also can be conducted to identify potential hazards.

Prevention

Once a job analysis is conducted and potential problems have been identified, prevention should be the next step. Prevention requires a thorough knowledge of the circumstances that surround environmental hazards as well as any predisposing biological or behavioral factors that may influence the capacity of a worker to perform the job in a safe and healthy manner.

Therefore, it is important to promote workplace education and awareness programs for the maintenance of musculoskeletal health and the prevention of injuries. Such programs can include education of workers, management, engineers, and support personnel in identifying sources of biomechanical stress and associated MSDs at the workplace.

Worker selection and placement

One of the preventive methods is the worker selection and placement process that selects and maintains a work force by using medical and/or performance criteria. The criteria identify individuals with health conditions or work capacities, such as reduced strength, that would increase their risk of personal injury if assigned to a job, and then place the workers in jobs accordingly.

However, it is important to identify high-risk jobs and quantify the required job demands to prevent abuse of such placement procedures. Workers should be matched with jobs that have specific demands and corresponding worker capacities. To do this, employers may have to use the skills of an ergonomist to evaluate job demands. Clinical experience in human physiology and performance assessment also may be needed for evaluating worker capacities.

Training

Training also may be used to control or prevent workplace injuries and illnesses. Training programs may range from basic instruction on the proper use of tools and materials, to instructions on emergency procedures and use of protective devices.

Detailed and specific training programs also can be developed and geared specifically toward worksite safety and health activities. Programs designed to broaden the worker's involvement include training in hazard identification (including observing and reporting hazards) and participating in facility-wide control programs.

The OSHA Training Institute in Illinois also offers courses that specifically deal with the major topics of ergonomics, including repetitive motion disorders, manual lifting and back injuries, vibration, temperature stress, and workstation design.

Tools, tasks, and workstation redesign

An important prevention method employs the principles of ergonomics to control workplace hazards through the redesign of work methods and tools.

Ergonomics takes into consideration the physiological, anatomical, and psychological capabilities and limitations of workers in relation to their work tasks, equipment used, and job environments. Ergonomics then tries to find the best fit between the human and the imposed job conditions to ensure and enhance worker health, safety, comfort, and productivity. The best fit usually is found by focusing on the job and tool redesign, rather than on worker training or selection.

Controlling workplace stress

According to OSHA, the ergonomic approach to workplace design is the most effective preventive measure and should be the first choice for controlling sources of workplace stress. Jobs and tools that are ergonomically redesigned are relatively permanent and, once implemented, do not normally require modification for each new employee.

Administrative controls such as employee selection and training may be considered secondary methods of control. Employee screening and selection methods can be subjective and discriminatory when considering which employees are considered fit for a particular job. Fitness for a job must be based on actual job demands that are often difficult to assess, and the general criteria of selecting only the strongest or the youngest workers should be avoided.

Also, training programs that require that each new employee be instructed and then monitored can be costly and less positive than engineering controls used as primary methods of prevention.

Ethylene oxide (1910.1047)

at a glance

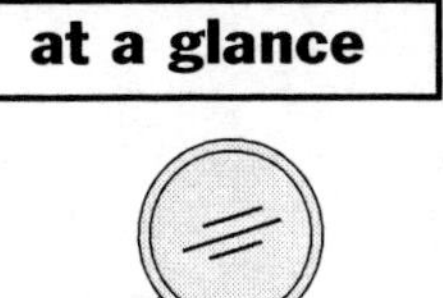

The ethylene oxide standard prevents exposures to ethylene oxide, a gas used as a chemical sterilant for heat-sensitive medical instruments.

EtO is a highly flammable, colorless gas with a distinctive sweet, ether-like odor that is detectable only at dangerously high levels of concentration in the air. EtO vapor is not usually detectable by scent until it reaches a concentration level of about 700 parts EtO per million parts of air (700 ppm), far above the PEL allowed by OSHA. Irritation of the eyes and upper respiratory system can occur at concentrations as low as 200 ppm. The high odor-detection threshold makes workplace monitoring and a gas-detection alarm system essential for protecting workers from the adverse effects of overexposure.

EtO commonly is used in laboratories and other healthcare facilities to sterilize heat- and moisture-sensitive medical instruments and equipment. Such sterilization usually is accomplished in an enclosed chamber, known as a sterilizer or autoclave, into which EtO is released from a gas cylinder or cartridge.

Unless good engineering controls and work practices are in place, workers who use sterilization equipment may encounter relatively high concentrations of EtO over brief periods. A special need exists to control short-term peak exposures, as might occur when a worker changes an EtO cylinder, opens a sterilization chamber door to unload it, transfers a sterilized load to an aerator, or reaches inside the chamber to clean it.

OSHA requirements

Employers are required to protect workers from exposure to EtO under the EtO standard.

The standard requires employers to determine whether worker exposure exceeds a specified action level of of 0.5 ppm calculated as an eight-hour TWA, and to institute work practices and engineering controls to keep exposure under the specified PELs.

The OSHA standard applies to all occupational exposure to EtO. However, an exemption exists for the processing, use, or handling of products that contain EtO if objective data show that the product cannot release the compound in airborne concentrations at or above the action level, and the product is not likely to release EtO in excess of the excursion limit during expected conditions of processing, use, or handling that will cause the greatest possible release. Employers are required to keep records to show that the products they use meet the exemption requirements.

OSHA PELs

OSHA requires employers to monitor worker exposure to EtO and institute controls to keep that exposure at or below PELs.

The PEL for EtO is an eight-hour TWA of 1 ppm with an excursion limit of 5 ppm for any 15-minute period. Employers that are subject to the EtO standard but fail to comply with its provisions may be subject to fines and other penalties authorized by the Occupational Safety and Health Act.

Written compliance plan

If employee exposure to EtO exceeds the TWA or excursion limit, the employer is required to establish and implement a written compliance plan to reduce exposure to within acceptable limits. The written plan must include a schedule for periodic leak-detection surveys and a plan for emergency situations.

Employee rotation is not permitted as a means of complying with the TWA or excursion limit.

Adverse health effects

High concentrations of EtO liquid or vapor can cause severe skin burns, rashes, sores, headache, nausea, and hemolysis, which is the destruction of red blood cells. Very high exposures may cause vomiting, shortness of breath, weakness, drowsiness, lack of coordination, cyanosis (bluish skin color resulting from oxygen insufficiency), and pulmonary edema.

Contact with EtO-sterilized equipment or wrappings that have not been adequately aerated to remove residual EtO may cause severe skin burns with large blisters and peeling skin. Healing may leave hyperpigmentation (i.e., brown discoloration of skin).

Long-term adverse health effects of EtO exposure include an increased risk of cancer and chromosomal damage. Adverse reproductive effects, such as spontaneous abortion, also may occur from EtO exposure.

Flammability

Typically, EtO is supplied in compressed gas cylinders that contain 88% chlorofluorocarbons and 12% ethylene oxide, a mixture that essentially renders it nonflammable. These cylinders generally are used with medium- or large-size sterilization units.

Pure EtO is marketed in single-dose cartridges that are used more often in smaller sterilization units. Although pure EtO may present a more serious fire hazard, it is thought to be safer in some ways because the single-dose cartridges are punctured inside the sterilization chamber, reducing the risk that workers could be inadvertently exposed to gas leaking from cylinders and external piping lines.

Monitoring

Environmental monitoring is required by OSHA under the EtO standard. Types of equipment used for such monitoring include the following:

- **Direct-reading instruments**—These devices, which include portable infrared analyzers, generally are used for area monitoring. The instruments may not be accurate at EtO concentrations below 1 ppm (1.8 mg/m^3) because they are sensitive to high humidity and can produce false readings.

- **Charcoal samples**—Activated charcoal tubes may be used to collect samples that are later analyzed to determine exposure for the entire sampling period, such as for an eight-hour day.

- **Passive dosimeters**—Usually worn on the worker's lapel, passive dosimeters can be chemically analyzed to provide a semi-quantitative indication of exposure.

Initial and periodic monitoring

OSHA requires all employers covered under the standard to conduct initial monitoring to determine accurately the airborne concentrations of EtO in the workplace to which employees may be exposed.

Determination of exposure must be made from breathing-zone air samples (not area samples) that are representative of the eight-hour TWA and 15-minute excursion limit exposure of each employee. Employee exposure is defined in the standard as exposure to EtO that would occur if the worker were not using respiratory-protective equipment. Generally, representative samples must be taken for each work shift in each job classification and work area where employees are exposed. However, if the employer can document that exposure levels are equivalent for similar operations in different work shifts, then exposure need only be determined for one shift.

If initial monitoring reveals that employee exposure to EtO is at or above the action level (0.5 ppm) but at or below the eight-hour TWA, the employer must conduct periodic monitoring for each such employee at least every six months; if exposure is above the eight-hour TWA, monitoring must occur at least every three months. This monitoring schedule may be altered from quarterly to semi-annually if the employee's exposure has decreased to or below the eight-hour TWA, as indicated by two consecutive measurements taken at least seven days apart.

If initial monitoring indicates that employee exposure is above the 15-minute excursion limit (5 ppm), the employer must conduct periodic monitoring at least every three months or as often as necessary to evaluate short-term exposure.

Termination of monitoring

TWA monitoring may be discontinued for certain employees if the initial monitoring reveals their exposure to be below the action level or if the periodic monitoring shows that exposures are below the action level in at least two consecutive measurements taken at least seven days apart.

Excursion-limit monitoring may be discontinued if the initial monitoring reveals employee exposure to be at or below the excursion limit or if periodic monitoring reveals employee exposures are at or below the excursion limit in at least two consecutive measurements taken at least seven days apart. If measurements indicate that exposure is below the action level, monitoring may be discontinued for those particular employees. If workplace processes or practices change in a manner that could cause new or additional exposure to EtO, monitoring must be resumed.

Examples of instances in which excursion-limit monitoring should be conducted include during cylinder changers, when opening the sterilizer door after completion of the sterilization cycle, and when the sterilized load is transferred to the aerator.

Monitoring accuracy

Monitoring required under the standard must be accurate (to a confidence level of 95%) to within +/- 25% for airborne concentrations of EtO at the 1 ppm level, and to within 35% for concentrations at the action level of 0.5 ppm.

Monitoring must be accurate (to a confidence level of 95%) to within +/- 35% for airborne concentrations of EtO at the excursion limit.

Employee notification

Employees must be notified of the results of the monitoring within 15 working days, either by written word on an individual basis or by appropriate posting. This notification must inform the employee as to what corrective action the employer is taking where exposure exceeds the PEL or the excursion limit.

Regulated areas

Employers must establish regulated areas wherever occupational exposures to EtO concentrations exceed or can reasonably be expected to exceed the excursion limit. These areas must be well marked and limited to authorized personnel.

Medical surveillance

Employers who are subject to the EtO standard are required to institute a medical surveillance program for all employees who are, or may be, exposed to EtO at or above the action level for at least 30 days a year, whether or not they use respirators.

Medical examinations and consultations must be made available without cost, without loss of pay, and at a reasonable time and place to employees as follows:

- Prior to assignment to an area where exposure may be at or above the action level for at least 30 days
- At least annually for each employee exposed at or above the action level for at least 30 days in the past year
- At termination of employment or reassignment to an area where exposure is not at or above the action level for at least 30 days a year
- As medically appropriate for any employee exposed during an emergency

- As soon as possible for an employee who either
  - notifies the employer of the development of signs or symptoms of overexposure
  - wants medical advice about the effects of current or past exposure on the individual's ability to produce a healthy child
- At frequencies determined by the examining physician when necessary

Medical exam content

Medical examinations required under the standard must include a medical and work history and physical examination with special emphasis on symptoms related to the pulmonary, hematologic, neurologic, and reproductive systems, and to the eyes and skin. The exam also must include

- a complete blood count that comprises at least a white cell count (including differential cell count), red cell count, hematocrit, and hemoglobin
- any laboratory or other test deemed necessary by the examining physician

Employees who show signs of overexposure or who desire information about their reproductive ability should have the content of their medical exam determined by the examining physician. The exam must include pregnancy testing or fertility evaluation if requested by the employee and deemed appropriate by the physician.

Information provided to physician

The employer is required to provide the following information to the examining physician:

- A copy of the EtO standard and appendices A, B, and C
- A description of the affected employee's duties as they relate to the exposure
- The employee's representative exposure level or anticipated exposure level

- A description of any PPE and respiratory equipment used or to be used
- Information from previous medical exams of the employee that would not otherwise be available to the physician

Physician's written opinion

The employer is required to obtain the examining physician's written opinion, which contains the results of the medical examination and all of the following:

- The physician's opinion as to whether the employee has any detected medical conditions that would place the employee at an increased risk of material health impairment from exposure to EtO
- Any recommended limitations on the employee or upon the use of PPE such as clothing and respirators
- A statement that the employee has been informed by the physician of the medical exam results and of any medical conditions that result from EtO exposure that require further explanation or treatment

The employer is required to instruct the physician not to reveal in the written opinion given to the employer any specific findings or diagnoses unrelated to occupational exposure to EtO. The written opinion must be provided to the employee within 15 days of its receipt by the employer.

Engineering and work practice controls

OSHA requires employers to institute engineering and work practice controls wherever feasible to reduce employee exposure to or below the PELs described in the standard.

Engineering controls are generally infeasible for collection of quality assurance sampling from sterilized materials, removal of biological indicators from sterilized materials, loading and unloading of tank cars, and vessel cleaning. For these operations, engineering controls are required only where OSHA demonstrates that such controls are feasible.

Engineering controls and design

OSHA recommends that laboratories and other healthcare facilities adopt workplace design modifications to better protect workers from exposure to EtO. Such modifications may include

- retrofitting sterilizers with an aeration cycle to eliminate exposure that occurs when transferring sterilized goods to a separate aerator unit.
- installation of gas line hand valves at the connection to the EtO supply cylinder to minimize leakage during cylinder change.
- installation of vented capture boxes in workplaces where the floor drain is located in the same room as the sterilizer or in a room where workers normally are present.
- ventilation of aeration units to a nonrecirculating or dedicated exhaust system and placement of the aerator unit as close as possible to the sterilizer to minimize exposure from the off-gassing of sterilized items as they are transferred to the aerator.
- ventilation controls that reduce the likelihood that workers will be exposed to short but high levels of EtO during cylinder change. Acceptable controls include
    - location of the cylinders in a well-ventilated room (under negative pressure) where workers are not usually present
    - installation of a flexible hose (where the sterilizer gas line is disconnected from the cylinder) to a nonrecirculating or dedicated exhaust system
    - installation of a hood (within one foot of where the cylinder change takes place) that is part of a nonrecirculating or dedicated exhaust system

- installation of a bleed valve that removes gas from the space between the tank valve and the charge valve; the bleed valve should discharge through a hose that is routed either to the capture box or directly to the dedicated exhaust system

- installation of a hood or metal canopy over the sterilizer doors to minimize worker exposure to EtO gas that may be released when the door is opened following the sterilization process. The hood or canopy must be connected to a nonrecirculating or dedicated exhaust system.

- ventilation of the sterilizer pressure-relief valves so that the valves exhaust vapor in one of the following ways:

  - Through a pipe connected to the outlet of the relief valve and ventilated directly outdoors at a point away from passersby and not near any windows or air intake vents
  - Through a connection to a nonrecirculating or dedicated exhaust system
  - Through a connection to a well-ventilated room where workers are not normally present

- installation of alarm systems to alert personnel of ventilation system failures, such as those that occur when the ventilation fan motor is not working.

Workplace practices

Workplace practices should be permanently posted near the door of each sterilizer. OSHA recommends the following workplace practices to control worker exposure to EtO:

- Supply line filters should be changed in the following manner:

  - Close the cylinder valve and the hose valve
  - Disconnect the cylinder hose from the cylinder
  - Open the hose valve and bleed slowly into a proper ventilating system
  - Vacate the area until the line is empty
  - Change the filter; reconnect the lines and reverse the value position
  - Check hoses, filters, and valves for leaks with a fluorocarbon leak detector (for sterilizers using the 12/88 EtO mixture)

- Because the used filter is likely to be saturated with EtO, industrial hygienists also recommend that the filter immediately be placed in a tightly sealable plastic bag (e.g., a Ziplock®) either to be aerated before disposal or disposed of as hazardous waste in accordance with federal and state laws and regulations.

- Restricted-access areas should exclude all personnel when certain operations are in progress, such as discharging a vacuum pump, emptying a sterilizer liquid line, or venting a nonpurge sterilizer with the door ajar.

- Doors of sterilizers with purge cycles should be opened immediately upon completion of the cycle, or the purge cycle should be repeated before opening.

- Doors of sterilizers without purge cycles should be left six inches ajar for 15 minutes and then fully ajar for another 15 minutes before the load is removed. If the level of exposure determined by peak monitoring for one hour after this time is above 10 ppm for an eight-hour TWA, more time should be added to the second waiting period.

- Procedures for unloading the chamber must include the use of baskets or rolling carts or tables to avoid excessive contact with materials and shorten worker exposure time. Carts should be pulled, not pushed, by workers to reduce off-gas exposure.

- A written maintenance log should be instituted to document the date of each leak detection and any maintenance performed.

- Leak detection should be performed on sterilizer door gaskets, cylinder and vacuum piping, hoses, filters, and valves, using full pressure with a fluorocarbon leak detector (for 12/88 systems) every two weeks. Cylinder piping connections should be checked after changing cylinders. The automatic solenoid valves that control EtO flow to the sterilizer should be checked.

- Maintenance personnel should replace sterilizer/aerator door gaskets, valves, and fittings when necessary as determined during biweekly checks; visual inspection for cracks, debris, and other foreign substances should be conducted daily by the operator.

Protective clothing and equipment

Where eye or skin contact with liquid EtO or EtO solutions might occur, OSHA requires employers covered under the standard to provide and ensure the use of proper protective equipment at no cost to the employee. Employers must make sure that protective clothing is impermeable to EtO.

OSHA recommends that workers should be provided with and required to wear protective clothing wherever there is significant potential for skin contact with liquid EtO solutions. Permeable clothing, including leather shoes and items made of rubber, should not be allowed to become contaminated with liquid EtO. If contamination occurs, such clothing should immediately be removed while the employee is under an emergency deluge shower. Contaminated leather footwear must be discarded.

Use of respirators

OSHA's EtO standard includes respiratory-protection provisions for employees who use respirators while performing EtO-related activities. Employers must provide the respirators and ensure that they are used during

- periods necessary to install or implement feasible engineering controls
- work operations, such as maintenance and repair activities, vessel cleaning, or other activities for which engineering and work practice controls are not feasible
- work operations for which feasible engineering and work practice controls are not yet sufficient to reduce employee exposures to or below the TWA
- emergencies

Respirator program

The employer must create a respiratory-protection program that meets applicable requirements of OSHA's respiratory-protection standard at 29 CFR 1910.134.

Respirator selection

Respirators used to meet the requirements of the standard must be among those approved as acceptable protection against EtO by NIOSH.

Respirators should be chosen according to the Table 1 at the end of this chapter.

Respirator fit testing

Under the respiratory-protection standard, before an employee may be required to use any respirator with a negative- or positive-pressure tight-fitting facepiece, the employee must be fit tested with the same make, model, style, and size of respirator to be used. Such employees must pass an appropriate qualitative or quantitative fit test prior to initial use of the respirator, whenever a different respirator facepiece is used, and at least annually thereafter. Additional fit tests may be required as necessary.

Additional requirements

The respiratory-protection standard also includes requirements for respirator use, maintenance, and care; breathing air quality and use; identification of filters, cartridges, and canisters; employee training and information; respirator program evaluation; employee medical evaluation; and recordkeeping.

Warning signs

The employer must post and maintain legible signs marking regulated areas and entrances or access ways to regulated areas. Such signs must bear the following legend:

DANGER
ETHYLENE OXIDE
CANCER HAZARD AND REPRODUCTIVE HAZARD
AUTHORIZED PERSONNEL ONLY
RESPIRATORS AND PROTECTIVE CLOTHING MAY BE REQUIRED
TO BE WORN IN THIS AREA

Warning labels

Precautionary labels must be put on all containers of EtO where the contents are capable of causing employee exposure at or above the action level or the excursion limit. The labels must remain on the containers that leave the workplace. The labels must comply with the requirements of OSHA's hazard communication standard and should contain the following legend:

DANGER
CONTAINS ETHYLENE OXIDE
CANCER HAZARD AND REPRODUCTIVE HAZARD

The label also must include a warning statement against breathing airborne concentrations of EtO.

Reaction vessels, storage tanks, and pipes or piping systems are not considered to be containers under the standard.

Material Safety Data Sheets (MSDSs)

Employers that manufacture or import EtO must comply with OSHA's hazard communication standard regarding the development of MSDSs.

Training and information

The employer must provide employees who are potentially exposed to EtO at or above the action level or above the excursion limit with information and training about EtO at the time of initial assignment and at least annually thereafter. According to the standard, employees should be informed of the following:

- The requirements of the EtO standard and an explanation of its contents, including material contained in Appendix A and B

- Any operations in their work area where EtO is present
- The location and availability of the written standard
- The medical surveillance program required under the standard and an explanation of the information contained in Appendix C

Employee training should include at least

- methods and observation that may be used to detect the presence or release of EtO in the work area (e.g., monitoring conducted by the employer, continuous monitoring devices, etc.)
- the physical and health hazards of EtO
- the measures employees can take to protect themselves from hazards associated with EtO exposure, including specific work practices, emergency procedures, and use of PPE required under the standard
- the details of the employer's hazard communication program, including an explanation of the labeling system and how employees can obtain and use hazard information

Exemption records

In cases where an employer seeks exemption from the standard's requirements because the product used is not capable of releasing EtO in airborne concentrations at or above the action level, the employer must keep records that include the following:

- The name of the product qualifying for the exemption
- The source of the objective data
- The testing protocol, results of testing, and/or analysis of the material for the release of EtO

- A description of the operation exempted and how the data support the exemption
- Other data relevant to the operations, materials, processing, or employee exposures covered by the exemption

Such records must be maintained for as long as the employer uses the product in the workplace and is exempted from the standard.

Exposure measurement records

Employers subject to the standard are required to keep accurate records of all measurements taken for the purpose of monitoring employee exposure to EtO. The record should contain at least the following information:

- The date of measurement
- The operation (work duties) that involves exposure to EtO that is being monitored
- Sampling and analytical methods used and evidence of their accuracy
- Number, duration, and results of samples taken
- Type of protective devices worn, if any
- Name, Social Security number, and any exposure encountered

Such records must be maintained for at least 30 years.

Medical surveillance records

Employers are required to establish and maintain an accurate record for each employee subject to medical surveillance under the standard. The medical record should include at least the following:

- The name and Social Security number of the employee
- Physician's written opinions

- Any employee medical complaints related to EtO exposure
- A copy of the information provided to the physician as required under the standard

Such records must be maintained for the duration of the individual's employment plus 30 years.

Availability of records

The employer must, upon written request, make all required records available for inspection and copying by OSHA. Exemption and exposure records must be made available for examination and copying to affected employees, former employees, and designated representatives in accordance with OSHA requirements for medical records. Employee medical records required under the standard must be made available for examination and copying to the subject employee and to anyone having the specific written consent of the employee.

Observation of monitoring

Employees and their designated representatives (e.g., union officials) must be provided with an opportunity to observe any monitoring of employee exposure to EtO conducted under the standard. When such observation requires entry into an area where the use of protective clothing or equipment is required, the observer should be provided with and be required to use the clothing or equipment and comply with all other applicable safety rules.

Table 1 **Minimum requirements for respiratory protection for airborne EtO**

Condition of use or concentration of airborne EtO (ppm)	Minimum required respirator
Equal to or less than 50	(a) Full-facepiece respirator with EtO-approved canister, front- or back-mounted.
Equal to or less than 2,000	(a) Positive-pressure supplied-air respirator, equipped with full facepiece, hood, or helmet, or (b) Continuous-flow supplied-air respirator (positive pressure) equipped with hood, helmet, or suit.
Concentration above 2,000 or unknown concentration (such as in emergencies)	(a) Positive-pressure SCBA, equipped with full facepiece, or (b) Positive-pressure full facepiece supplied-air respirator equipped with an auxiliary positive-pressure SCBA.
Firefighting	(a) Positive-pressure SCBA equipped with full facepiece.
Escape	(a) Any respirator described above.
Note: Respirators approved for use in higher concentrations are permitted to be used in lower concentrations.	

Exiting (1910.36)

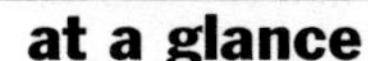

at a glance

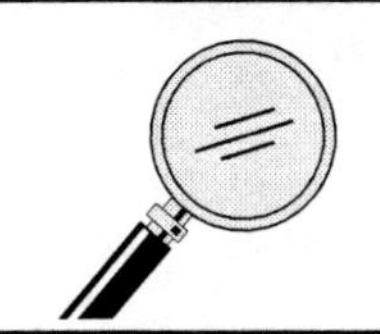

OSHA requires every building designed for human occupancy to provide exits that permit prompt escape in an emergency. OSHA's requirements also include 1910.155 to 1910.165, which are part of the fire-prevention standards.

Every building designed for human occupancy shall be provided with exits sufficient to permit the prompt escape of occupants in case of emergency (29 CFR 1910.36).

Every building or structure must be provided with exits of kinds, numbers, locations, and capacities appropriate to the individual building or structure, with regard to occupancy, number of persons exposed, fire protection available, and height and type of construction of the building or structure (29 CFR 1910.36[b]).

Exits, and the way to and from exits, must be unobstructed and accessible at all times (29 CFR 1910.37[a][3]).

All exits must let out directly to the street or other open space that gives safe access to a public way (29 CFR 1910.36[c][1]).

Exit doors that serve more than 50 people, or at high-hazard areas, must swing in the direction of exit travel (29 CFR 1910.36[e][2]).

Exits must be marked by readily visible, suitably illuminated exit signs that are distinctive in color and contrast with their surroundings. The word "EXIT" must be in plainly legible letters, not less than six inches high (29 CFR 1910.37[b][2], [6], and [7]).

Any door, passage, or stairway that is neither an exit nor a way of exit access, and that is located so that it can be mistaken for an exit, must be identified by a sign reading "Not an Exit" or similar designation (29 CFR 1910.37[b][5]).

In hazardous areas, or where employees may be endangered by the blocking of any single means of exit due to fire or smoke, there shall be at least two means of exit remote from each other.

An employer who complies with NFPA code 101, the *Life Safety Code™*, 2000 edition, will be deemed to be compliant with the corresponding requirements in 29 CFR 1910.34, 36, and 37 (29 CFR 1910.35).

Eye/face protection (1910.133 and various standards)

at a glance

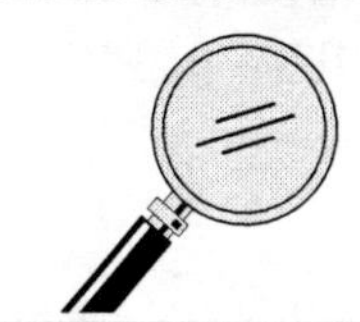

The eye and face protection standard sets requirements for protecting the eyes and faces of workers.

Appropriate eye or face protection is required wherever there is a possibility of injury from flying particles, molten metal, liquid chemicals, acids or caustic liquids, chemical gases or vapors, or potentially injurious light radiation (29 CFR 1910.133).

Employees must use eye protection that provides side protection when there is a hazard from flying objects. Detachable side protectors (e.g., clip-on or slide-on side shields) are acceptable.

For protection from injurious light radiation, equipment must have filter lenses that have a shade number appropriate for the work being performed.

Employees who wear prescription lenses are required to wear eye protection that either incorporates the prescription in the design or can be worn over the prescription lenses without disturbing their proper position (e.g., goggles).

OSHA also requires that eye and face protection meet performance standards developed by ANSI. The following specifics apply:

- If purchased after July 5, 1994, devices must comply with ANSI standard Z87.1-1989, "American National Standard Practice for Occupational and Educational Eye and Face Protection"
- If purchased before July 5, 1994, devices must comply with ANSI standard Z87.1-1968, "USA Standard for Occupational and Educational Eye and Face Protection"

Eye and face protection must be clearly marked for easy identification of the manufacturer.

Examples of work duties that might require eye and/or face protection include use of machinery that produces dust and chips, handling of toxic and corrosive substances, processes that can produce aerosols of infectious agents, gas or electrical welding, and medical-equipment sterilization. Supervisors and visitors to the work area also must wear required protective gear.

Eyewash/emergency shower (1910.151)

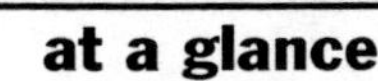

at a glance

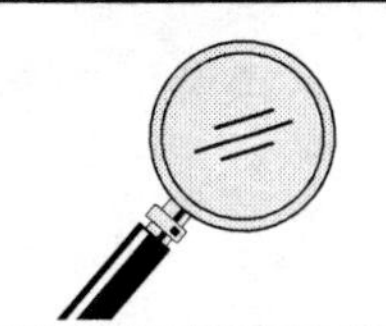

OSHA has some requirements related to eyewash stations and emergency showers in its medical first aid standard, although in interpretation letters it points to a well-known ANSI standard.

Suitable facilities for quick drenching or flushing of the eyes and body shall be provided within the work area for immediate emergency use if there is a possibility that an employee might be exposed to injurious, corrosive materials (29 CFR 1910.151[c]).

Employers must provide showers for those employees who work in areas where they are exposed above the PELs or who work in regulated areas, so they may shower at the end of their shift. For employees who work at a hazardous waste clean-up site that will be in operation for six months or more, showers are to be provided for their use at the end of the work shift (29 CFR 1910.120[n][7] and 1910.1018[m][2]).

Fire prevention and protection (1910.155 to 1910.165)

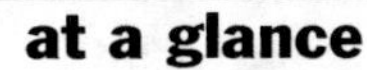

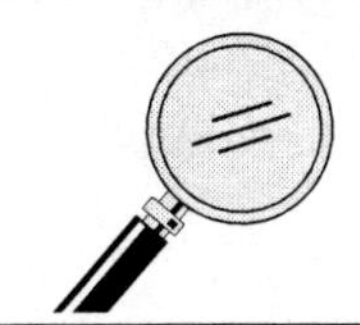

The fire protection standard sets requirements for exits, extinguishers, and fire brigades.

OSHA imposes standards (Subpart L—29 CFR 1910.155–1910.165) that require employers to take fire-protection precautions. Employers should be certain that all materials are stored, handled, and stacked with due respect for their fire-hazard characteristics. Significant quantities of hazardous materials must be separated from the main bulk of storage by fire walls. Regarding exit routes, employers have the option of adopting the NFPA's *LSC* (NFPA 101) version 2000 instead of the OSHA standard (29 CFR 1910.34–37).

OSHA's fire-protection standard applies to all places of employment except for maritime, construction, and agriculture. The standard contains requirements for fire brigades, all portable and fixed fire-suppression equipment, fire-detection systems, and fire or employee alarm systems installed to meet OSHA requirements.

Employee emergency-action and fire-prevention plans

When required by a specific OSHA standard, both a written emergency-action plan and a fire-prevention plan must be developed, kept in the workplace, and made available to employees for review. Employers with 10 or fewer employees can communicate the plans orally and need not maintain a written plan. OSHA imposes specific requirements for the contents of such plans (29 CFR 1910.38).

Emergency-action plan

The emergency-action plan should include, at a minimum, the following elements:

- The preferred means and procedures for reporting fires and other emergencies

- Emergency-escape procedures, types of evacuation, and emergency-exit-route assignments
- Procedures to be followed by employees who remain to operate critical plant operations before evacuation
- Procedures to account for all employees after emergency evacuation is complete
- Assigned rescue or medical duties
- The name or title of every employee who may be contacted by coworkers who need either more information about the plan or an explanation of their duties under the plan

Employers also must maintain an employee alarm system that uses distinct signals for each purpose. Employers must designate and train employees to assist in the safe and orderly evacuation of other employees. The plan must be reviewed with employees when the plan is developed, when an employee is initially assigned to a job affected by the plan, when the employee's responsibilities under the plan change, or when the plan is changed.

Facilities should be aware of related emergency-action-planning requirements under the OSHA formaldehyde standard (29 CFR 1910.1047) and EtO standard (29 CFR 1910.1048). Emergency-planning requirements under the OSHA HAZWOPER standard (29 CFR 1910.120), while not directed specifically at events involving fires, also may dovetail with the OSHA fire-protection standard mandates.

Fire-prevention plan

The fire-prevention plan should include the following elements:

- A list of the major workplace fire hazards and their proper handling and storage procedures, potential ignition sources and their control procedures, and the type of fire-protection equipment or systems that can control each major hazard
- Procedures to control accumulations of flammable and combustible waste

- Names or job titles of the personnel responsible for maintenance of fire-prevention equipment and systems
- Names or job titles of personnel responsible for controlling fuel-source hazards
- Provisions to ensure that employees are trained in the particular procedures of the plan for which each is responsible

The employer should properly maintain fire-control equipment and systems installed on heat-producing equipment to prevent accidental ignition of combustible equipment. Also, all fire-alarm signaling systems should be maintained and tested in accordance with OSHA standards.

Fire brigades

The OSHA fire-protection standard imposes specific requirements that employers must follow if they establish a fire brigade (29 CFR 1910.156). Maintaining such a brigade essentially means that the facility runs its own fire department. Because of the extensive preparation, training, staffing, and equipment requirements to maintain a fire brigade, laboratory facilities normally choose not to establish one. Rather, they rely on local fire departments to respond to fire emergencies at the facility.

When establishing a facility fire brigade, the employer is first required to prepare and maintain a written organizational policy that explains the structure of the brigade, the type and amount of training to be provided, and the size and expected duties of the brigade. The policy must be made available for OSHA inspectors and for employees or their representatives.

Employees who are expected to perform interior structural firefighting should be physically capable of performing any assigned emergency duties. Any employee with known heart disease, epilepsy, or emphysema should not be permitted to participate in fire-brigade emergencies without a physician's certificate. The employer must provide employees who perform interior structural firefighting with personal protective clothing at no cost to the employee.

Training

All fire-brigade members should have training that is commensurate with their responsibilities and that occurs at least annually. Fire-brigade members who are expected to perform interior structural firefighting should have at least quarterly training. The quality of the training should be similar to that received at state- or university-operated professional training schools. Fire-brigade members should be informed about special hazards such as the presence of flammable liquids and gases, toxic chemicals, radioactive sources, and water-reactive substances to which they may be exposed during a fire. They should be notified of any changes in hazards and should be trained in special precautions to be taken to address these hazards.

Firefighting equipment

Firefighting equipment must be maintained and inspected at least annually to ensure safe operability. Portable fire extinguishers and respirators must be inspected monthly. Damaged or unserviceable equipment must be removed and replaced.

Protective clothing

The employer must provide to employees who perform interior structural firefighting appropriate protective clothing at no cost. Such clothing is not required for those who use only fire extinguishers or standpipe systems to control small fires.

When protective clothing is required, it must meet specific standards of performance and construction specified in the fire-protection standard. The clothing in combination must completely protect the head, body, and extremities, and must consist of the following:

- **Foot and leg protection.** Protective footwear, such as fully extended boots or boots and trousers in a combination that is water- and slip-resistant, must be provided.

- **Body protection.** Body protection should be coordinated with foot and leg protection to ensure full body protection for the wearer. It must meet applicable NFPA standards for performance, construction, and fire resistance.

- **Hand protection.** Gloves must protect against cuts, punctures, and heat penetration. They must meet NIOSH criteria for firefighters' gloves.

- **Eye, face, and head protection.** Head protection must meet U.S. Fire Administration criteria for performance of firefighters' helmets. Eye and face protection must be used when hazards of flying or falling materials are present.

Respiratory protection

OSHA's respiratory-protection standard (29 CFR 1910.134) addresses the use of respirators in IDLH atmospheres, including interior structural firefighting. The standard requires that during interior structural firefighting SCBA must be used, and two firefighters must be on standby to provide assistance or perform rescue when two firefighters are inside a burning building.

Employers must ensure that respirators are provided to, and used by, fire-brigade members. The respirators must meet requirements of the respiratory-protection standard. SCBA must have a minimum service-life rating of 30 minutes in accordance with NIOSH specifications under 42 CFR 84, except for self-contained breathing apparatuses used only for emergency-escape purposes.

The buddy system

NFPA recognizes that firefighters must operate in teams of two or more when conducting interior structural firefighting operations. OSHA has clarified that failure to respond with teams of two or more is a violation of OSHA's general duty clause.

The respiratory-protection standard and industry practice as codified through the NFPA standards require that a minimum of four firefighters be involved in emergency operations during interior structural firefighting. Two people must serve as a team in the hazardous area, and two must stand by outside the area to monitor the operation and provide assistance if a rescue is necessary.

Firefighters who work in teams of two or more (i.e., using the buddy system) in IDLH atmospheres are required to maintain communications by voice, visual contact, or tethering with a signal line. Radio or electronic contact cannot be substituted for direct visual contact.

Portable fire extinguishers

The fire-protection standard imposes certain requirements when employers provide portable fire extinguishers for use in the workplace (29 CFR 1910.157).

In general, only approved fire extinguishers should be used, and they must be readily and safely accessible at all times. Extinguishers that contain carbon tetrachloride or chlorobromomethane extinguishing agents should not be used. Extinguishers should be selected based on the classes of anticipated workplace fires (classes A–D) and on the size and degree of hazard that may occur.

Distribution

Extinguishers should be placed so that maximum travel distances, unless there are extremely hazardous conditions, do not exceed 75 feet for class A extinguishers or 50 feet for class B. Employers with written emergency action plans that meet the standard's requirements are exempt from distribution requirements for portable extinguishers.

Uniformly spaced standpipe systems or hose stations connected to a sprinkler system may be used instead of class A portable fire extinguishers, provided that such systems meet requirements and employees are trained at least annually on their use.

Inspection, maintenance, and testing

Portable fire extinguishers must be maintained in fully charged and operable condition at all times. Portable fire extinguishers must be visually inspected monthly and have an annual maintenance check. The annual maintenance date should be recorded and the record retained for either one year after the last entry or the life of the shell, whichever is shorter.

Hydrostatic testing

All portable fire extinguishers must be hydrostatically tested at intervals specified in the standard. Such testing is also required after an extinguisher is repaired, damaged, corroded, or otherwise compromised.

All soldered- or riveted-shell, self-generating soda acid, self-generating foam, or gas cartridge water–type portable fire extinguishers that are operated by inverting the extinguisher to rupture the cartridge or initiate an uncontrollable pressure-generating chemical reaction to expel the agent should be permanently removed from service.

Training

When portable extinguishers are provided, employees who may use them must be trained in their use and the hazards involved in the early stages of firefighting. The training should be provided initially upon hiring and annually thereafter.

Standpipe and hose systems

The OSHA standard imposes requirements on Class II and III standpipe and hose systems, which are designed for use by employees rather than by professional firefighters (29 CFR 1910.158). The systems must be located and protected appropriately to prevent mechanical damage. Damaged standpipes must be repaired promptly.

Equipment

Fire-hose reels or cabinets must be designed for prompt use of the hose valves, hose, and other equipment during an emergency. The reels and cabinets should be conspicuously identified and used only for fire equipment.

Hose outlets and connections should be located high enough above the floor to avoid being obstructed yet remain accessible to employees. Appropriate adapters must be provided throughout the system to ensure that the hose connections are compatible with those used on the supporting fire equipment.

A hose should be of such length that friction loss resulting from water flowing through the hose will not decrease the pressure at the nozzle below 30 psi. Standpipe hoses must be equipped with shutoff-type nozzles.

Water supply

The minimum water supply for standpipe and hose systems should be sufficient to provide 100 gallons per minute for a period of at least 30 minutes.

Testing and maintenance

The piping of Class II and Class III systems, including yard piping, must be hydrostatically tested. Hose on all standpipe systems must be hydrostatically tested with couplings in place.

The hose system must be properly maintained. Water-supply tanks must be filled to the proper level. Proper pressure must be maintained where pressure tanks are used.

The hose system should be inspected at least annually and after each use to ensure that the equipment and hose are in place, available for use, and serviceable. Hemp or linen hose on existing systems should be unracked, inspected, and reracked using a different fold pattern at least annually. When the system or any portion is found not to be serviceable, it should be removed from service immediately and replaced with equivalent protection, such as extinguishers and fire watches.

Trained persons should be appointed to conduct all required inspections.

Automatic-sprinkler systems

Automatic-sprinkler systems must meet specific requirements under the fire-protection standard (29 CFR 1910.159). Systems installed to meet OSHA requirements prior to 1981 are acceptable, provided that they comply with NFPA or National Board of Fire Underwriters standards in effect at the time of the systems' installation.

All automatic sprinkler designs must provide the necessary discharge patterns, densities, and water-flow characteristics for complete coverage in a particular workplace or zoned subdivision of the workplace. The employer must maintain the automatic-sprinkler system and ensure that a main-drain flow test is performed on each system annually. The employer also must conduct acceptance tests as specified by OSHA and record the test dates.

Every automatic-sprinkler system must be provided with at least one automatic water supply capable of providing design water flow for at least 30 minutes. An auxiliary water supply or equivalent protection should be provided when the automatic water supply is out of service, except for systems of 20 or fewer sprinklers. The employer may attach hose connections for firefighting use to wet-pipe sprinkler systems, provided that the water supply satisfies the combined design demand for sprinklers and standpipes.

Piping should be protected against freezing and corrosion. All dry-sprinkler pipes and fittings should be installed so that the system can be totally drained.

Only approved sprinklers may be used. A local waterflow alarm must be provided on all sprinkler systems that have more than 20 sprinklers. Sprinklers must be placed to provide the maximum area of protection per sprinkler. The minimum vertical clearance between sprinklers and material in the area below the sprinklers should be 18 inches.

Hydraulically designed automatic-sprinkler systems must be identified according to the design of the system. Central records may be used in lieu of signs at sprinkler valves, provided that the records are available for inspection and copying by OSHA inspectors.

Fixed extinguishing systems

The OSHA fire protection standard requires that all fixed extinguishing system components and agents be approved for use on the specific fire hazards they are expected to control (29 CFR 1910.160). Fixed extinguishing systems using dry chemicals, gaseous agents, water spray, or foam must comply with OSHA requirements.

Alarm systems must be provided to indicate when the system is discharging. Discharge alarms are not required on systems where discharge is immediately recognizable.

Employees must be warned against entry into discharge areas where the atmosphere is hazardous to employee safety or health. Warning or caution signs should be posted either at the entrance to or inside of areas protected by fixed extinguishing systems that use agents in concentrations known to be hazardous.

Fixed extinguishing systems must be inspected annually. The weight and pressure of refillable containers should be checked semiannually. Factory-charged nonrefillable containers that have no means of pressure indication should be weighed semiannually. Inspection and maintenance dates must be recorded either on the container or in a central location. A record of the last semi-annual check must be kept until the container is checked again, or for the life of the container, whichever is shorter.

The employer must train designated employees to inspect, maintain, operate, or repair fixed extinguishing systems. Annual refresher training also must be provided.

Chlorobromomethane or carbon tetrachloride may not be used as an extinguishing agent when employees may be exposed.

Automatic-detection equipment must be installed and maintained in accordance with OSHA standards.

At least one manual station must be provided for discharge activation of each fixed extinguishing system. The manual operating devices should be identified according to the hazard against which they will provide protection.

PPE must be used for immediate rescue of employees trapped in hazardous atmospheres.

Total flooding systems

The employer must provide an appropriate emergency-action plan for each workplace area protected by a total flooding system that provides agent concentrations exceeding maximum safe levels. On all total flooding systems, a predischarge alarm that meets requirements and gives employees time to safely exit from the discharge area prior to system discharge must be provided.

The employer must provide automatic actuation of total flooding systems by means of an approved fire-detection device installed and interconnected with a predischarge employee alarm system.

Dry-chemical systems

Employers must ensure that dry chemicals in such systems are compatible with other foams or wetting agents that may be used. Different types of dry chemical agents must not be mixed, and the system must be sampled for effectiveness at least annually. An alarm that provides ample warning for employees to evacuate must be sounded if dry chemicals that may obscure vision are used. Designed extinguishing levels must be reached in 30 seconds (29 CFR 1910.161).

Gaseous-agent systems

Designed concentrations of gaseous agents must be maintained until the fire is extinguished or controlled. Precautions must be taken to prevent employee exposure to toxic levels of the agents. Designed extinguishing concentrations must be reached in 30 seconds, or in 10 seconds for Halon systems. An alarm system must be set up to ensure that employees are warned to evacuate before unsafe concentrations of any agent are reached (29 CFR 1910.62).

Water-spray and foam systems

Such systems must be effective in controlling fire in protected areas. System drainage should be directed away from areas where employees are working and away from emergency egress (29 CFR 1910.63).

Fire-detection systems

Fire-detection equipment should be approved for the purpose for which it is intended under the OSHA standard (29 CFR 1910.164). All detection systems should be restored to proper operating condition as soon as possible after each test or alarm. Spare detecting devices and components that are normally destroyed in the process of detecting fires should be available for prompt restoration of the system.

Maintenance and testing

Fire-detection systems and fire detectors should be tested and adjusted as often as needed to maintain proper reliability and operating condition. Factory-calibrated detectors need not be adjusted after installation.

Pneumatic and hydraulically operated detection systems installed after January 1, 1981, must be equipped with supervised systems. The object of supervision is detection of any failure of the circuitry, and the employer should use any method that will ensure that the system's circuits are operational.

Electrically operated sensors for air pressure, fluid pressure, or electrical circuits can provide effective monitoring and are the typical types of supervision.

Maintenance and testing, including cleaning and necessary sensitivity adjustments, must be performed by an appropriately trained individual. Cleaning necessary to remove dust or other particulates should be done at regular intervals.

Protection of detectors

Fire detectors must be protected from corrosion as well as from mechanical or physical impact that might make them inoperable. Detectors must be supported independently of their attachment to wires or tubing.

Response time

Fire-detection systems installed to actuate fire extinguishment or suppression systems must be designed to operate in time to control a fire.

Fire-detection systems installed to speed up employee alarm and evacuation must provide a warning for emergency action and safe escape.

Alarms or devices initiated by fire-detector actuation must not be delayed for more than 30 seconds unless the delay is necessary for the immediate protection of employees. If such a delay is necessary, it should be noted in the emergency-action plan.

Number, location, and spacing

The number, location, and spacing of detectors should be based on design data. This information can be obtained from the approval listing for detectors or from NFPA standards. It also can be obtained from fire-protection engineers or manufacturers of fire-detection systems.

Employee alarm systems

Under the OSHA standard, the employee alarm system must provide warning for necessary emergency action as called for in the emergency-action plan, provide reaction time for safe escape of employees from the workplace, or do both (29 CFR 1910.165).

The employee alarm must be perceived above ambient noise or light levels by all employees in the affected portion of the workplace. Tactile devices may be used to alert employees who would not otherwise be able to recognize the audible or visual alarm. The alarm must be distinctive and recognizable as an alarm to evacuate the work area or perform actions designated under the emergency-action plan.

The employer should explain to each employee the preferred means for reporting emergencies, such as manual pull-box alarms, public address systems, radios, or telephones. Emergency telephone numbers should be posted near telephones, employee notice boards, and other conspicuous places when telephones serve as a means of reporting emergencies. Emergency messages should have top priority.

The employer should establish procedures for sounding emergency alarms in the workplace. If there are 10 or fewer employees, voice communication is acceptable provided all employees can hear the call. These workplaces need not have a backup system.

Installation and restoration

All devices, components, or systems used must be approved under the OSHA fire-protection standard. Steam whistles, air horns, strobe lights or similar lighting devices, or tactile devices that meet OSHA requirements are considered acceptable.

Maintenance and testing

Nonsupervised employee alarm systems must be tested for reliability every two months. Backup means of alarm, such as employee runners or telephones, must be provided when systems are out of service for testing or other reasons.

Employee alarm circuitry installed after January 1, 1981, should be supervised so that it will provide positive notice to personnel whenever a deficiency exists in the system. Supervised alarm systems must be tested at least annually.

All servicing, testing, and maintenance must be done by trained personnel. Manually operated actuation devices for use in conjunction with employee alarms must be unobstructed, conspicuous, and readily accessible.

Formaldehyde (1910.1048)

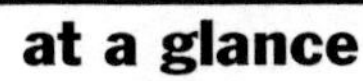

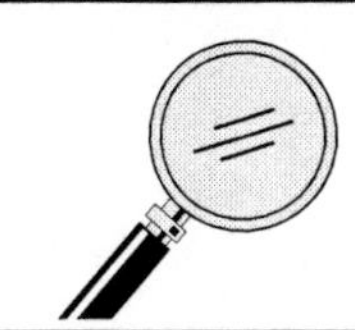

at a glance

The formaldehyde standard limits exposures to formaldehyde, which is used in laboratories as a disinfectant and tissue preservative.

Formaldehyde is a colorless, pungent gas that can be detected by scent at air concentrations of less than 1 ppm. Formaldehyde is also supplied commercially in a liquid solution, known as formalin, which contains alcohol or water.

Occupational exposure to formaldehyde vapor or liquid can cause adverse health effects that range from mild to life-threatening. A particular danger associated with formaldehyde is that some workers develop olfactory fatigue (i.e., they lose their ability to detect formaldehyde in the air, except at dangerously high concentrations).

In laboratory facilities, formaldehyde is utilized primarily as a disinfectant or a tissue preservative. Employees at risk of exposure include those who work in histology and pathology laboratories.

Adverse health effects

Formaldehyde is a known carcinogen. Exposure may result in an increased risk of cancer in the nose, sinuses, and lungs. Other adverse health effects can be caused by direct contact with liquid formaldehyde or inhalation of the vapor, as follows:

- **Inhalation**—Formaldehyde is highly irritating to the upper airways. Vapor concentrations above 50 ppm can cause severe pulmonary reactions, including pulmonary edema, pneumonia, and bronchial irritation that can result in death. Formaldehyde also can cause lower-airway irritation characterized by coughing, wheezing, and chest tightness. Some controversy exists over whether formaldehyde gas can cause occupational asthma.

- **Eye contact**—Eyes may burn, itch, become red, and tear from exposure to formaldehyde vapor. Accidental splashes of liquid formaldehyde can cause corneal damage and blindness.

- **Skin contact**—Skin contact with liquid formaldehyde can result in irritation, contact dermatitis, and sensitization. Symptoms include erythema (abnormal redness), edema, and vesiculation or hives.

- **Ingestion**—Ingestion of formaldehyde can cause nausea, vomiting, severe abdominal pain, and death.

OSHA standard

The OSHA formaldehyde standard applies to all occupational exposure to formaldehyde, including formaldehyde gas and solutions and material products that release the substance.

The standard requires employers to determine whether worker exposure exceeds a specified action level of 0.5 ppm calculated as an eight-hour TWA, and to institute work-practice and engineering controls to keep exposure below specified PELs.

An exemption to the standard's monitoring requirements is allowed in cases where the employer documents, using objective data, that the presence of formaldehyde in the workplace cannot result in airborne concentrations that would cause any employee to be exposed at or above the action level or the STEL under foreseeable conditions of use.

PELs

Employees may not be exposed to airborne concentrations of formaldehyde that exceed either 0.75 ppm as an eight-hour TWA or 2 ppm as a 15-minute STEL.

Exposure monitoring

The OSHA standard requires employers to conduct monitoring for employees who may be occupationally exposed to formaldehyde to determine the extent of their exposure. Such employee exposure is defined as that which would occur without use of a respirator.

Tools used to determine formaldehyde exposure levels include personal dosimeters, industrial hygiene wet methods that use detector tubes, and impingers with a solution of sodium bisulfite.

Written compliance plan

If exposure monitoring indicates that employee exposure is over either PEL, the employer is required to develop and carry out a written plan to reduce employee exposure and to give written notice to employees. The written notice must contain a description of the corrective action being taken to decrease exposure.

Regulated areas

Regulated areas must be established where the concentration of airborne formaldehyde exceeds either the TWA or the STEL. All entrances and access ways must be posted with warning signs. Signs must bear the following information:

DANGER
FORMALDEHYDE
IRRITANT AND POTENTIAL CANCER HAZARD
AUTHORIZED PERSONNEL ONLY

Access to regulated areas must be limited to authorized persons who have been trained to recognize the hazards of formaldehyde. Both the access restrictions applicable to established regulated areas at a multi-employer work site and the locations of these areas must be communicated to other employers that are working there.

Monitoring

The standard requires employers to identify all employees who may be exposed to formaldehyde at or above the action level or the STEL. The exposure level of each such employee then must be accurately determined.

A representative sampling strategy may be developed in cases where an employer chooses not to measure the exposure of each individual covered under the standard. Such a strategy should measure sufficient exposures within each job classification for each work shift to correctly characterize and not underestimate the exposure of any employee within each exposure group. Representative sampling measurements must denote the employee's full shift or short-term exposure to formaldehyde, as appropriate. Representative samples for each job classification in each work area must be taken for each shift unless it can be documented with objective data that exposure levels for a given job classification are equivalent for different work shifts.

Initial monitoring

Initial monitoring must be repeated each time there is a change in production, equipment, process, personnel, or control measures that may result in new or additional exposure to formaldehyde.

Periodic monitoring

The standard requires employers to periodically monitor employees for whom initial monitoring indicates that they are exposed at or above the action level or the STEL. If results reveal employee exposure to be at or above the action level, monitoring must be repeated at least every six months. If those results reveal employee exposure at or above the STEL, monitoring must be repeated at least annually under worst conditions.

Periodic monitoring may be discontinued for employees if results from two consecutive sampling periods taken at least seven days apart show that employee exposure is below the action level and the STEL. The results must be consistent with the employer's knowledge of the job and work operation.

Monitoring accuracy

OSHA requires that exposure monitoring be accurate, at the 95% confidence level, to within +/- 25% for airborne concentrations of formaldehyde at the TWA and the STEL and to within +/- 35% for airborne concentrations of formaldehyde at the action level.

Employee notification

Employers must notify employees of the results of exposure monitoring within 15 days of receiving them. Notification should be given in writing, either by distributing copies of the results to the employees or by posting the results.

Observation

Affected employees or their designated representatives must be provided with the opportunity to observe any monitoring of employee exposure to formaldehyde required by this standard. When such observation means that the observer must enter an area where the use of protective clothing or equipment is required, the clothing and equipment must be provided to the observer, and measures must be taken to ensure that it is used by the observer. In addition, the observer must comply with all other applicable safety and health procedures.

Engineering and work-practice controls

OSHA requires employers to institute engineering and work-practice controls to reduce and maintain employee exposures to formaldehyde at or below the TWA and the STEL. However, if it has been established that feasible engineering and work-practice controls cannot reduce employee exposure to or below either of the PELs, these controls must be applied to reduce employee exposures to the extent feasible, and they must be supplemented with respirators that satisfy the requirements of the standard.

Respirator selection and use

The formaldehyde standard includes respiratory-protection provisions for employees who wear respirators while performing formaldehyde-related activities. Employers must provide the respirators and ensure that they are used during

- periods necessary to install or carry out feasible engineering and work-practice controls
- work operations, such as maintenance and repair activities or vessel cleaning, for which the employer establishes that engineering and work-practice controls are not feasible
- work operations for which feasible engineering and work-practice controls are not yet sufficient to reduce exposure to or below the PEL
- emergencies

Respirator program

Whenever respirator use is required, employers must create a respiratory-protection program that meets applicable requirements of OSHA's respiratory-protection standard (29 CFR 1910.134).

If air-purifying chemical-cartridge respirators are used, unless the cartridge contains a NIOSH-approved ESLI to show when breakthrough occurs, the employer must replace

- the cartridge after three hours of use or at the end of the work shift, whichever occurs first
- canisters used in atmospheres up to 7.5 ppm (10 x PEL) every four hours and industrial-sized canisters used in atmospheres up to 75 ppm (100 x PEL) every two hours, or at the end of the work shift, whichever occurs first

Respirator selection

The employer must select appropriate NIOSH-approved respirators as specified in Table 1 at the end of this chapter.

A powered air-purifying respirator must be made available to any employee who experiences difficulty wearing a negative-pressure respirator to reduce exposure to formaldehyde.

Respirator fit testing

Under the respiratory-protection standard, before an employee may be required to use any respirator with a negative- or positive-pressure tight-fitting facepiece, the employee must be fit tested with the same make, model, style, and size of respirator to be used. Such employees must pass an appropriate qualitative or quantitative fit test prior to initial use of the respirator, whenever a different respirator facepiece is used, and at least annually thereafter. Additional fit tests may be required as necessary.

Additional requirements

The respiratory-protection standard also includes requirements for respirator use, maintenance, and care; breathing air quality and use; identification of filters, cartridges, and canisters; employee training and information; respirator program evaluation; employee medical evaluation; and recordkeeping.

PPE and clothing

Employers are required to provide employees covered under the standard with appropriate PPE and clothing in accordance with OSHA's standard on PPE. Specifically, the employer must comply with that standard's general requirements (29 CFR 1910.132) and provisions for eye and face protection (29 CFR 1910.133).

Required protective equipment or clothing must be provided to employees at no cost. Employers must ensure that employees wear them. OSHA also states the following:

- Protective equipment and clothing should be selected based upon the form of formaldehyde to be encountered, the conditions of use, and the hazard to be prevented.

- Chemical protective clothing made of material impervious to formaldehyde must be used to prevent all contact of liquids containing 1% or more formaldehyde to the eyes and skin. PPE, such as goggles and face shields, must be used as appropriate to the operation. Contact with irritating or sensitizing materials must be prevented to the extent necessary to eliminate the hazard.

- Where face shields are worn, chemical safety goggles also are required if there is a danger of formaldehyde reaching the area of the eyes.

- Full-body protection must be worn for entry into areas where concentrations exceed 100 ppm and for emergency reentry into areas of unknown concentration.

Laundry and ventilation

Protective equipment and clothing that has become contaminated with formaldehyde must be cleaned or laundered before its reuse.

When ventilating formaldehyde-contaminated clothing and equipment, a storage area must be established so that employee exposure is minimized. Containers for contaminated clothing and equipment and storage areas must have labels and signs that state

DANGER
FORMALDEHYDE-CONTAMINATED (CLOTHING) EQUIPMENT
AVOID INHALATION AND SKIN CONTACT

Only persons trained to recognize the hazards of formaldehyde may be allowed to remove the contaminated material from the storage area for purposes of cleaning, laundering, or disposal. Any person who launders, cleans, or repairs such clothing or equipment must be informed of formaldehyde's potentially harmful effects and of procedures to safely handle the clothing and equipment.

The employer must ensure that employees do not take home equipment or clothing that is contaminated with formaldehyde.

All required protective clothing and equipment must be repaired or replaced for each affected employee as necessary to ensure its effectiveness.

Hygiene facilities

Clean and sanitary change rooms must be provided for employees who are required to change from work clothing into protective clothing to prevent skin contact with formaldehyde. The change rooms should comply with OSHA sanitation requirements.

Conveniently located quick-drench showers also must be provided if employees' skin may become splashed with solutions that contain 1% or greater formaldehyde (e.g., because of equipment failure or improper work practices). Assurance must be made that affected employees use these facilities immediately.

Acceptable eyewash facilities within the immediate work area for emergency use must be provided if there is any possibility that an employee's eyes may be splashed with solutions that contain 0.1% or greater formaldehyde.

Preventive maintenance and housekeeping

A program to detect leaks and spills, including regular visual inspections, must be conducted for operations involving formaldehyde liquids or gas.

Preventive maintenance of equipment, including surveys for leaks, must be performed regularly.

In work areas where spillage may occur, provisions to contain the spill, decontaminate the work area, and dispose of the waste must be made. Assurance must be made that all leaks are repaired and spills are cleaned promptly by employees who wear suitable protective equipment and are trained in proper methods of cleanup and decontamination.

Formaldehyde-contaminated waste and debris that results from leaks or spills must be placed for disposal in sealed containers that bear a label warning of formaldehyde's presence and the hazards associated with formaldehyde.

Emergencies

Appropriate procedures are adopted to minimize injury and loss of life for each workplace where there is the possibility of an emergency involving formaldehyde. Appropriate procedures must be carried out in the event of an emergency.

Medical surveillance

Under the formaldehyde standard, medical surveillance programs must be instituted for the following workers:

- All employees exposed to formaldehyde at concentrations at or exceeding the action level or exceeding the STEL
- Any employees who develop signs and symptoms of overexposure to formaldehyde
- Any employees exposed to formaldehyde in emergencies

When determining whether an employee may be experiencing signs and symptoms of possible overexposure, look to signs and symptoms associated with formaldehyde exposure that occur only in exceptional circumstances when airborne exposure is less than 0.1 ppm and when formaldehyde is present in materials in concentrations less than 0.1%.

Medical surveillance procedures

All medical procedures, including administration of medical disease questionnaires, must be performed by or under the supervision of a licensed physician. They must be provided without cost to the employee, without loss of pay, and at a reasonable time and place.

Medical surveillance must be made available to employees prior to assignment to a job where formaldehyde exposure is at or above the action level or above the STEL and annually thereafter.

The surveillance should be made available promptly upon determining that an employee is experiencing signs and symptoms indicative of possible overexposure to formaldehyde. It should include

- administration of a medical disease questionnaire, which is designed to elicit information about work history, and evidence of eye, nose, or throat irritation; chronic airway problems or hyperreactive airway disease; allergic skin conditions or dermatitis; and upper- or lower-respiratory problems.

- a determination of whether a medical examination is necessary for employees who are not required to wear respirators to reduce formaldehyde exposure. This determination must be made by the physician and based on evaluation of the medical disease questionnaire.

Medical examinations

Medical examinations must be given to any employee who the physician feels, based on information in the medical disease questionnaire, may be at increased risk from exposure to formaldehyde.

These examinations also must be given at the time of initial assignment and at least annually thereafter to all employees required to wear a respirator to reduce exposure to formaldehyde. The medical examination must include the following:

- A physical examination with emphasis on evidence of irritation or sensitization of the skin and respiratory system, shortness of breath, or irritation of the eyes.

- Laboratory examinations for respirator wearers that consists of baseline and annual pulmonary function tests. As a minimum, these tests must consist of forced vital capacity, forced expiratory volume in one second, and forced expiratory flow.

- Any other test the examining physician deems necessary to complete the written opinion.

- Counseling of employees who have medical conditions that would be directly or indirectly aggravated by exposure to formaldehyde on the increased risk of impairment of their health.

Employees who have been exposed to formaldehyde in an emergency should have medical exams made available as soon as possible. The examination must include a medical and work history with emphasis on any evidence of upper- or lower-respiratory problems, allergic conditions, skin reaction or hypersensitivity, and any evidence of eye, nose, or throat irritation. Other examinations must consist of those elements considered appropriate by the examining physician.

Information provided to physician

The following information must be provided to the examining physician:

- A copy of the standard and appendices A, C, and D
- A description of the affected employee's job duties as they relate to the employee's exposure to formaldehyde
- The representative exposure level for the employee's job assignment
- Information concerning any PPE and respiratory protection used or to be used by the employee
- Information from previous medical examinations of the affected employee within the control of the employer
- In the event of a nonroutine examination because of an emergency, the physician must be provided as soon as possible with a description of how the emergency occurred and the exposure the victim may have received

The physician's written opinion

The examining physician's written opinion must be obtained for each examination required under the standard. This written opinion must contain the results of the medical examination, but it may not reveal specific findings or diagnoses unrelated to occupational exposure to formaldehyde. The written opinion must include the following:

- The physician's opinion as to whether the employee has any medical condition that would place the employee at an increased risk of material impairment of health from exposure to formaldehyde

- Any recommended limitations on the employee's exposure or changes in the use of PPE, including respirators

- A statement that the employee has been informed by the physician of any medical conditions that would be aggravated by exposure to formaldehyde, whether these conditions may have resulted from past formaldehyde exposure or from exposure in an emergency, and whether there is a need for further examination or treatment

Retention of the results of the medical examination and tests conducted by the physician must be provided.

A copy of the physician's written opinion must be provided to the affected employee within 15 days of its receipt.

Medical removal

The formaldehyde standard generally requires employers to remove workers who experience certain adverse health effects due to formaldehyde exposure from positions where they are exposed and reassign them to other job duties.

The medical removal provisions apply when an employee reports significant irritation of the mucosa of the eyes or the upper airways, respiratory sensitization, dermal irritation, or dermal sensitization attributed to workplace formaldehyde exposure.

Medical removal provisions do not apply in the case of dermal irritation or dermal sensitization when the product suspected of causing the dermal conditions contains less than 0.05% formaldehyde.

Basic requirements

When symptoms of possible overexposure are reported, the condition should be evaluated by a physician selected by the employer. A two-week observation period must follow, and if the condition worsens and the physician finds that significant irritation resulting from workplace formaldehyde exposure is present, the physician may recommend restrictions or removal of the employee from a particular work area.

Under the standard, the employer is required to comply promptly with the restrictions or recommendation of the physician and remove the affected employee from the current formaldehyde exposure. If possible, the employee should be transferred to comparable work for which the employee is qualified or can be trained in a short period of time (up to six months). When an employee is removed under these provisions, the formaldehyde exposure in the new environment must be as low as possible and no greater than the action level.

The removed employee's current earnings, seniority, and other benefits must be maintained. Within six months after removal, an examining physician must determine whether the affected employee can return to the original job status or if the removal is to be permanent.

Second medical opinion

After the employer selects the initial physician who conducts any medical examination or consultation to determine whether an employee should be removed, the employee may designate a second physician to review the findings.

If the second review differs from the first, the employee or authorized employee representative may designate a third physician to render an opinion. The recommendation of the third physician will be binding on the employer unless the employee and the employer reach an agreement that is otherwise consistent with the recommendations of at least one of the three physicians.

Hazard communication

For purposes of hazard communication, formaldehyde gas, all mixtures or solutions composed of greater than 0.1% formaldehyde, and materials capable of releasing formaldehyde into the air under any normal condition of use at concentrations reaching or exceeding 0.1 ppm must be considered a health hazard. Specific health hazards that must be addressed include cancer, irritation and sensitization of the skin and respiratory system, eye and throat irritation, and acute toxicity.

MSDSs

Any employer who uses formaldehyde-containing materials that constitute a health hazard as defined in the standard must comply with the requirements of the section that pertain to MSDSs in the hazard-communication standard. Manufacturers, importers, and distributors of formaldehyde-containing materials that constitute a health hazard as defined in the standard must ensure that MSDSs and updated information are provided to all employers who purchase such materials at the time of the initial shipment and at the time of the first shipment after the MSDS is updated.

Labels

Labels must be placed on all materials capable of releasing formaldehyde at levels of 0.1 ppm to 0.5 ppm. The labels should identify that the product contains formaldehyde, list the name and address of the responsible party, and state that the physical and health hazard information is readily available from the employer and from MSDSs.

For materials capable of releasing formaldehyde at levels above 0.5 ppm, labels must appropriately address all hazards as defined in appendices A and B of the hazard-communication standard, including respiratory sensitization. The labels must contain the words "potential cancer hazard."

Manufacturers and importers who produce or import formaldehyde or formaldehyde-containing products must provide downstream employers that use or handle these products with an objective determination through the required labels and MSDSs if these items may constitute a health hazard within the meaning of hazard determination under normal conditions of use.

Written communication plan

A written hazard-communication program must be developed and maintained at the workplace for formaldehyde exposure in the workplace. The program, at a minimum, must describe how the requirements for labels and other forms of warning, MSDSs, and employee information and training will be met.

Alternative warning labels

The use of warning labels required by other statutes, regulations, or ordinances that impart the same information as the warning statements required under these regulations also may be used.

Training

The formaldehyde standard requires employers to ensure that all employees who are assigned to workplaces where there is a health hazard from formaldehyde participate in a training program.

Employees must be provided with information and training on formaldehyde at the time of their initial assignment and whenever a new hazard from formaldehyde is introduced into their work area, unless the employer can show that employees are not exposed to formaldehyde at or above 0.1 ppm. This information and training must be provided at least annually.

The training program must be conducted in a manner that the employee is able to understand. It must include the following:

- A discussion of the contents of this regulation and contents of the MSDS.
- The purpose for and description of the medical surveillance program required by this standard, including a description of the potential health hazards associated with exposure to formaldehyde and a description of the signs and symptoms of exposure to formaldehyde. Instructions to immediately report to the employer the development of any adverse signs or symptoms that the employee suspects are attributable to formaldehyde exposure must be given.

- A description of operations in the work area where formaldehyde is present and an explanation of the safe work practices appropriate for limiting exposure to formaldehyde in each job.
- The purpose for, proper use of, and limitations of personal protective clothing and equipment.
- Instructions for the handling of spills, emergencies, and clean-up procedures.
- An explanation of the importance of engineering and work-practice controls for employee protection and any necessary instruction in the use of these controls.
- A review of emergency procedures, including the specific duties or assignments of each employee in the event of an emergency.

The location of written training materials must be provided to affected employees and must be made readily available, free of cost.

Upon request, all training materials relating to the employee training program must be provided to OSHA and NIOSH.

Exposure monitoring records

An accurate record of all measurements taken to monitor employee exposure to formaldehyde must be established and maintained. This record must include the following information:

- The date of measurement
- The operation to be monitored
- The methods of sampling and analysis and evidence of their accuracy and precision
- The number, durations, times, and results of samples taken

- The types of protective devices worn
- The names, job classifications, Social Security numbers, and exposure estimates of the employees whose exposures are represented by the actual monitoring results

When the standard does not require monitoring, maintain a record to emphasize and prove that employees are not exposed to formaldehyde at or above the action level.

Medical surveillance records

An accurate record for each employee subject to medical surveillance under this standard must be established and maintained. This record must include the following information:

- The name and Social Security number of the employee
- The physician's written opinion
- A list of any employee health complaints that may be related to exposure to formaldehyde
- A copy of the medical examination results, including medical disease questionnaires and results of any medical tests required by the standard or mandated by the examining physician

Respirator records

Accurate records for employees subject to negative-pressure respirator fit testing must be established and maintained. This record must include the following information:

- A copy of the protocol selected for respirator fit testing
- A copy of the results of any fit testing performed

- The size and manufacturer of the types of respirators available for selection
- The date of the most recent fit testing, the name and Social Security number of each tested employee, and the respirator type and facepiece selected

Records retention

Any records required by the standard must be retained for at least the following periods:

- Exposure records and determinations must be kept for at least 30 years
- Medical records must be kept for the duration of employment plus 30 years
- Respirator fit testing records must be kept until replaced by a more recent record

Records availability

Upon request, all records maintained as a requirement of this standard must be made available to OSHA and NIOSH. Employee exposure records, including estimates made from representative monitoring, must be made available upon request for examination and copying to the subject employee, or former employee, and employee representatives in accordance with OSHA requirements on employee access to medical records.

Employee medical records required by this standard must be provided upon request for examination and copying to the subject employee or former employee, or to anyone having the specific written consent of the subject employee or former employee.

Table 1

Minimum requirements for respiratory protection against formaldehyde

Condition of use or formaldehyde concentration (ppm)	Minimum required respirator[1]
Up to 7.5 ppm (10 x PEL)	Full facepiece with cartridges or canisters specifically approved for protection against formaldehyde.[2]
Up to 75 ppm (100 x PEL)	Full-face mask, chest, or back-mounted type, with industrial-size canister specifically approved for protection against formaldehyde. Type C supplied-air respirator, demand type, with full facepiece, hood, or helmet.
Above 75 ppm or unknown (emergencies) (100 x PEL)	SCBA with positive-pressure full facepiece. Combination supplied-air, full-facepiece positive-pressure respirator with auxiliary self-contained air supply.
Firefighting	SCBA with positive-pressure in full facepiece.
Escape	SCBA in demand or pressure-demand mode. Full-face mask with chin style or front- or back-mounted type with industrial-size canister specifically approved for protection against formaldehyde.

Note:

1. Respirators specified for use at higher concentrations may be used at lower concentrations.
2. A half-mask respirator with cartridges specifically approved for protection against formaldehyde can be substituted for the full-facepiece respirator provided that effective gas-proof goggles are provided and used in combination with the half-mask respirator.

General duty clause

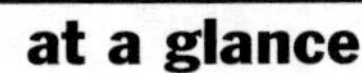
at a glance

The general duty clause requires employers to keep a workplace free of hazards that cause or may cause death or serious physical harm. Citations also may be linked to specific standards.

In the course of an OSHA survey, if an inspector identifies a serious workplace hazard not covered under a specific standard, the inspector may issue a citation based on Section 5(a)(1) of the Occupational Safety and Health Act, also known as the general duty clause. The clause states: "Each employer must furnish to each of his employees employment and a place of employment which are free from recognized hazards that are causing or likely to cause death or serious physical harm to his employees" (Public Law 91-596).

The purpose of the general duty clause is to provide a forum for the enforcement of fundamental safety practices, thus initiating the requirement for employers to establish and maintain a workplace free from hazards that cause or may cause death or serious physical harm. Citations received under the general duty clause also may be linked to specific related standards, depending on the hazards identified.

General duty clause violations

OSHA may categorize a violation of the general duty clause as either a serious violation, a willful violation, or a repeated violation. OSHA will not issue a nonserious general duty clause violation. To issue a general duty clause violation, the following conditions must exist:

- Employees were exposed to a hazard because the employer failed to keep the workplace free of the hazard
- The hazard was recognized based on industrial or employer recognition, or "common sense"
- The hazard was causing or was likely to cause death or serious physical harm
- There was a feasible and useful method to correct the hazard

General duty clause restrictions

OSHA may not issue a general duty clause violation when another specific standard applies to a hazard, although the agency may cite it in the alternative when a standard is cited but it is unclear whether the standard applies. In addition, OSHA may not use the general duty clause to

- impose a requirement(s) that is more strict than a standard
- require an abatement method(s) that is not required under a standard
- enforce a "should" clause(s) in a standard
- cover categories of hazards that are exempted by a standard

Violations in healthcare facilities

Because of the "catch-all" nature of the general duty clause, violations are possible in any physical location of a healthcare facility. General duty clause violations issued in healthcare facilities during 2005 included the following:

- Employee sustained injury due to the collapse of boxes containing records. The boxes had been placed at a height greater than the employee's height, and no portable ladder or other appropriate device was available.

- Employees were exposed to tuberculosis through unprotected contact with a patient suspected of the infection and later confirmed to be infectious.

- The eyewash station provided in a location where employees used gluteraldehyde as a cold sterilization procedure did not have a water flow sufficient to flush both eyes simultaneously.

Other general duty clause violations covered topics such as burns, electric, falls, machine guarding, crushing, and chemical hazards.

The OSHA guidelines include workplace violence and ergonomics as possible general duty clause violations. See the related chapters for more information.

Glutaraldehyde

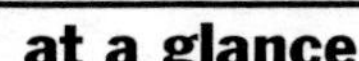

at a glance

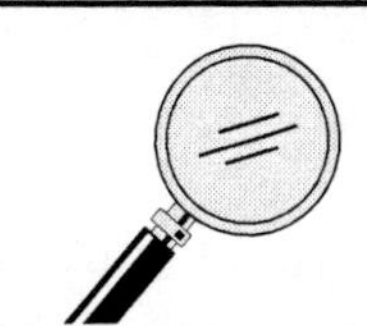

Glutaraldehyde is primarily a disinfectant for cold sterilization of medical instruments. OSHA tried to enforce an exposure limit under revisions to the air contaminants standard but failed.

Glutaraldehyde is used in laboratories as a disinfectant. Pathology and histology labs use glutaraldehyde as a tissue fixative. As a disinfectant, glutaraldehyde is used in a solution to sterilize table tops.

Adverse effects such as eye, nose, and throat irritation have been reported at air concentrations as low as 0.3 ppm. The odor threshold for glutaraldehyde is 0.04 ppm. Vapor concentrations as high as 20 ppm can be generated at room temperature (68° F) by solutions of 50% or more.

Glutaraldehyde solutions

Glutaraldehyde is available for use in various concentrations. In the laboratory, glutaraldehyde is used as a fixative in much stronger concentrations (e.g., solutions of 20%, 50%, and 99% glutaraldehyde).

Glutaraldehyde solutions may contain surfactants to promote rinsing, sodium nitrite to inhibit corrosion, peppermint oil as an odorant, and dyes that indicate activation of the solution. Buffered solutions generally are unstable and must be dated and replaced every two to four weeks.

Products that contain glutaraldehyde include Cidex, Wavicide, Metricide, and Omnicide.

Adverse health effects

Glutaraldehyde is absorbed into the body by inhalation, skin contact, and ingestion. It is irritating to the skin and mucous membranes at concentrations of about 0.3 ppm (1.05 mg/m^3). Even incidental or occasional occupational exposure can cause allergic contact dermatitis. Extensive skin contact may cause allergic eczema and may affect the nervous system.

Workers exposed to glutaraldehyde have reported ill effects that include eye, throat, and lung irritation; coughing; chest tightness; headaches; skin irritation; and asthma-like symptoms. Animal studies have shown a link between glutaraldehyde and fetotoxicity and chromosomal damage.

Exposure limits

An exposure limit ceiling of 0.2 ppm (0.8 mg/m^3) for glutaraldehyde is recommended by NIOSH. The ACGIH recommends a more stringent threshold limit value ceiling of 0.05 ppm (0.2 mg/m^3).

OSHA's air contaminants standard does not list a PEL for glutaraldehyde. However, OSHA adopted a ceiling limit of 0.2 ppm despite a failed regulatory attempt. OSHA has indicated that it may use the general duty clause of the Occupational Safety and Health Act to authorize enforcement action against employers that fail to provide employees with a level of protection supported by current data on adverse health effects. For this reason, many safety and health experts advise employers to monitor and institute controls to meet the 0.2 ppm ceiling.

Monitoring devices

Air sampling for glutaraldehyde may be accomplished by using personal monitoring badges and direct-reading instruments.

Ventilation controls

Glutaraldehyde overexposure is most likely to occur in poorly ventilated rooms. Employers should ensure that their ventilation systems are adequate. Some experts recommend a minimum of six air changes per hour. However, the American Institute of Architects recommends that soiled workrooms should have a minimum of 10 air changes per hour.

Proper ventilation is most critical in situations where the chemical is kept in large vats or trays. Local-exhaust ventilation and fume hoods generally are suggested for these areas.

Work practices and PPE

Exposure to glutaraldehyde vapor and liquid may occur when large containers of the chemical are left uncovered, accidentally spilled, or emptied out to drain. Therefore, vats, trays, and other open containers of glutaraldehyde should be kept covered whenever possible and tightly closed when not in use.

To prevent skin contact, employees should wear PPE, including splash-proof goggles and/or face shields, gloves, impermeable aprons, and other protective clothing as needed. Gloves should be made of a material that is impervious to glutaraldehyde (e.g., butyl, nitrile, or vinyl rubber).

An OSHA letter of interpretation on latex-glove use with glutaraldehyde says double gloving with latex gloves is suggested only if none of the above-mentioned gloves is available. OSHA's letter cites tests on latex gloves against glutaraldehyde that show breakthrough in 45 minutes. Therefore, latex gloves—if they are used—should be used only in cases of short-term, incidental contact. In addition, the gloves need to be changed often (i.e., every 10 to 15 minutes) and disposed of properly.

Employees also should be instructed to immediately wash or shower skin that becomes contaminated with glutaraldehyde. Eyewash stations and quick-drench showers may be provided for that purpose. Avoid breathing glutaraldehyde vapors. Promptly remove contaminated clothing and do not rewear it until the glutaraldehyde has been removed. Place the soaking container near a sink so that the employee will not have to carry the container across the room. Laboratories should check first with local regulations regarding disposal of glutaraldehyde into sanitary sewers.

Respiratory protection is considered a last line of defense where glutaraldehyde fumes cannot be brought below the 0.05 ppm exposure limit recommended by ACGIH.

Spill procedures

Employers should have a written procedure for cleaning up incidental spills of glutaraldehyde, and employees should be trained to follow the procedures and use PPE properly.

OSHA and best practices

OSHA has published *Best Practices for the Safe Use of Glutaraldehyde in Health Care*, a 48-page document educating healthcare employers and employees about exposure to glutaraldehyde. The document contains recommendations applicable to all healthcare settings on

- selection and use of personal protective equipment
- employee information and training
- exposure monitoring
- disposal of glutaraldehyde solutions
- spill control and cleanup procedures

Best Practices is available at *www.osha.gov/Publications/glutaraldehyde.pdf.*

Hazard communication standard (29 CFR 1910.1200)

at a glance

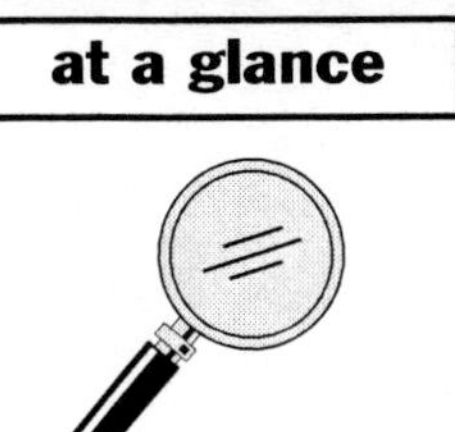

The standard consistently ranks among those most frequently cited as a result of a laboratory facility inspection. It requires employers to inform employees of potential health hazards associated with exposure to chemicals used or stored in the workplace.

The purpose of the hazard communication standard is to ensure that the hazards of all chemicals used in the workplace are evaluated by manufacturers and that this information is transmitted to employers who, in turn, must provide the information to employees. The transmittal of information to employees should be accomplished through a comprehensive hazard communication program that includes use of labels and other forms of warning, MSDSs, and employee training.

Generally, the hazard communication standard applies to any chemical used in the workplace. However, OSHA has issued full and partial exemptions covering, for example, "normal use" of consumer products in the workplace, laboratory work covered by OSHA's laboratory safety standard, and warehouse workers and other employees who handle chemicals only in sealed containers.

Chemicals covered

The hazard communication standard applies to any chemical that is known to be present in the workplace and to which employees could be exposed under normal conditions of use or in a foreseeable emergency.

General chemical exemptions

The hazard communication standard's requirements do not apply to certain types of chemical substances. Exempt substances include

- drugs that are packaged by the manufacturer for sale to consumers in a retail establishment (e.g., over-the-counter drugs) and drugs intended for personal consumption by employees in the workplace (e.g., first-aid supplies). This exemption does not cover powder, aerosol, or liquid prescription drugs.

- hazardous wastes that are regulated by the EPA under the RCRA or the CERCLA. The CERCLA exemption applies to any hazardous substance as defined by the law when the hazardous substance is the focus of remedial or removal action being conducted under CERCLA in accordance with EPA regulations. It is OSHA's intent to exempt CERCLA-listed chemicals only in circumstances where they are fully regulated by EPA, making OSHA's hazard communication standard requirements duplicative.

- consumer products or manufactured items that do not release more than minute or trace amounts of a hazardous chemical and that do not pose a physical hazard or health risk to employees. The normal use of consumer products in the workplace will not result in citations. According to OSHA inspection guidelines, citations will be issued only when the use of the product is inconsistent with the manufacturer's intentions or the frequency of use or duration of use greatly exceeds that expected of an ordinary consumer. OSHA compliance officers who issue citations for either consumer products or manufactured items must describe the specific hazardous chemical in the product, and the citation must name the specific chemical.

Partial exemption for laboratories

Most on-site hospital laboratories are subject to hazard communication requirements under a separate OSHA rule for occupational exposure to hazardous chemicals in laboratories.

The laboratory standard (29 CFR 1910.1450) contains provisions that preempt certain hazard communication standard requirements. For example, labs that are required by the other standard to have a written chemical hygiene plan need not comply with the hazard communication rule's written plan requirements.

The hazard communication rule does, however, require laboratories that are subject to the laboratory standard to

- ensure that labels on incoming containers of hazardous chemicals are not removed or defaced
- keep MSDSs that are received with incoming shipments of hazardous chemicals and make them readily accessible to laboratory employees
- ensure that employees are provided with information and training as required under the hazard communication standard

Laboratories not covered under the separate standard are responsible for full compliance with the hazard communication standard.

Partial exemptions to labeling requirements

The hazard communication standard's labeling requirements do not apply to certain items already covered under other federal labeling requirements. These include

- consumer products subject to the labeling requirements of the Consumer Product Safety Commission
- chemical substances or mixtures subject to labeling requirements of the Toxic Substances Control Act and labeling regulations issued under the act by the EPA
- pesticides subject to labeling requirements imposed by the EPA

Partial exemption where employees handle sealed containers

In work operations where employees only handle chemicals in sealed containers, employers are exempt from certain provisions and required only to

- ensure that labels on incoming containers of hazardous chemicals are not removed or defaced
- maintain copies of any MSDSs that are received with incoming shipments of sealed containers
- obtain an MSDS for any hazardous chemical received without one if an employee so requests
- ensure that MSDSs are readily accessible to employees during each work shift
- provide employees with information and training to the extent necessary to protect them in the event of a hazardous chemical spill or leak

Hazard communication program elements

Employers that are not producers or importers of chemicals generally need only focus their efforts on complying with provisions related to establishing a workplace hazard communication program, according to OSHA. These include requirements for

- a written plan
- labeling and hazard warnings
- maintenance and availability of MSDSs
- employee information and training

Written program

Employers covered by the standard are required to develop and maintain a written hazard communication program. At a minimum, the written program must

- describe how the standard's provisions for container labeling, MSDSs, and employee training will be met in that employer's workplace
- list the hazardous chemicals in each work area
- explain methods that will be used to inform employees of hazards involved in nonroutine tasks (e.g., periodic cleaning of equipment) and hazards associated with chemicals contained in unlabeled pipes in their work areas

The written hazard communication program must be available, upon request, to employees, their designated representatives, OSHA, and NIOSH.

Where employees must travel between workplaces during a workshift (i.e., their work is carried out at more than one geographical location), the written hazard communication program may be kept at the primary workplace facility.

Written program for multi-employer work sites

Additional written program requirements apply to employers that operate at multi-employer work sites (i.e., where employees of more than one employer are working).

Specifically, the standard requires employers that produce, use, or store hazardous chemicals in a way that employees of other employers might be exposed to them to ensure that their written hazard communication program covers the methods

- that will be used to provide the other employers with on-site access to MSDSs for each hazardous chemical to which their employees may be exposed while working

- the employer will use to inform the other employers of any precautionary measures that need to be taken to protect employees during normal work operations and in the event of a foreseeable emergency

- the employer will use to inform the other employers of the labeling system in use

Container labels and other written warnings

The employer must ensure that each container of hazardous chemicals in the workplace is labeled or marked with information that includes

- the identity of the hazardous chemical

- appropriate hazard warnings or, alternatively, words, pictures, and/or symbols that provide at least general hazard information and that, in conjunction with other information immediately available to employees under the program, will provide specific information regarding physical and health hazards of the chemical

Stationary process containers

The employer may use signs, placards, process sheets, batch tickets, operating procedures, or other such written materials in lieu of affixing labels to individual stationary process containers, as long as the material identifies the containers to which it is applicable and contains the required information. The written materials must be readily accessible to employees in their work areas throughout each work shift.

Employers need not label portable containers into which hazardous chemicals are transferred from labeled containers and that are intended only for the immediate use of the employee who performs the transfer.

The standard also specifies that employers

- may not deface or remove existing labels on incoming containers unless the containers are immediately marked with the required information.

- must ensure that labels and other written warnings are legible, in English, and prominently displayed on the container or readily available in the work area throughout each shift. Warning information may be in a language other than English where appropriate, as long as the information is presented in English as well.

- need not affix new labels to comply with these requirements, if existing labels already convey the required information.

- revise the labels within three months of becoming aware of significant information regarding the hazards of a chemical. Labels on containers shipped after that time should contain the new information.

Where a hazardous chemical is regulated by a substance-specific OSHA standard, the employer must ensure that the labels or other forms of warning used are in accordance with the requirements of that standard.

Employee information and training

Employers are required to provide employees with information and training on hazardous chemicals in their work area

- at the time of their initial assignment
- whenever a new hazard is introduced into their work area

Information and training may be designed to cover categories of hazards (e.g., flammability, carcinogenicity) or specific chemicals. Chemical-specific information must always be available, however, through labels and MSDSs.

Information

Employees must be informed of the requirements of the standard, any operations in their work area where hazardous chemicals are present, and the location and availability of the written hazard communication program. This includes the required list of hazardous chemicals and MSDSs.

Training

Employee training must include at least

- methods and observations that may be used to detect the presence or release of hazardous chemicals
- the physical and health hazards in the work area
- measures employees may take to protect themselves from these hazards, including specific procedures the employer has implemented to protect employees from hazardous exposure (e.g., work practices, PPE, etc.)
- the details of the employer's hazard communication program, including an explanation of the labeling system, MSDSs, and how employees can obtain and use the available hazard information

Employers are responsible for obtaining and maintaining an MSDS for each hazardous chemical that is used in their workplace.

MSDSs

Employers are required to

- maintain an MSDS for each hazardous chemical used in the workplace
- ensure that these MSDSs are readily accessible during each work shift to employees when they are in their work areas

If employees must travel between workplaces during a workshift, MSDSs can be kept at a central location at the primary workplace facility. However, the employer must ensure that employees can immediately obtain the required information in an emergency.

MSDSs may be kept in any form (including operating procedures) and may be designed to cover groups of hazardous chemicals (e.g., in a work area where it is more appropriate to address hazards of a process rather than individual chemicals) as long as the employer ensures that the required information is provided for each chemical and is readily accessible in the work area during each shift.

Electronic access to MSDSs

In the inspection guidelines, OSHA clarifies that employers may provide MSDSs to employees through computers, microfiche machines, the Internet, CD-ROMs, and fax machines. Employers that use electronic means must ensure that

- reliable devices are readily available in the workplace at all times
- workers are trained in the use of these devices, including specific software
- there is an adequate backup system in the event of the failure of that system, such as power outages or online access delays
- the system is part of the overall hazard communication program of the workplace

Employees must be able to access hard copies of the MSDSs, and in medical emergencies, employers must be able to immediately provide copies of the MSDSs to medical personnel.

Employee exposure records

Certain chemical identification information contained in MSDSs may have to be retained for 30 years as part of an employee's chemical exposure records under OSHA employee exposure and medical record access regulations (29 CFR 1910.20). However, these regulations stipulate that the MSDSs themselves need not be retained for any specified period as long as some record of the identity of the chemical, where it was used, and when it was used is retained for at least 30 years.

MSDSs must be available upon request to designated employee representatives, OSHA, and NIOSH.

Hazard determination and other requirements

The hazard communication standard requires chemical manufacturers, importers, and, in some cases, retail distributors to comply with additional provisions. These include requirements for assessing health and physical hazards of chemical products and supplying employers with up-to-date and accurate information on container labels and MSDSs.

Employers that choose to conduct their own hazard assessments on chemicals or chemical mixtures also may be subject to many of these requirements.

Container labeling

Chemical manufacturers, importers, and distributors are required to provide hazard information with delivery of hazardous chemicals. Each container must be labeled, tagged, or marked with the following information:

- Identity of the hazardous chemical(s)
- Appropriate hazard warnings
- The name and address of the chemical manufacturer, importer, or responsible party

MSDSs

Chemical manufacturers and importers must develop and supply an MSDS for each chemical to the receiving employer at the time of initial shipment. Retail distributors that sell hazardous chemicals also must provide an MSDS upon request.

New information about health or physical hazards must be incorporated on the MSDS within three months following the manufacturer's receipt of the information. The new MSDS must be transmitted to the employer with the next shipment of the chemical. Information must be in English, and include at least

- the identity of the chemical used on the label, unless it qualifies as a trade secret

- chemical and common names for the hazardous chemical

- information about the physical and chemical characteristics of the hazardous chemical, known acute and chronic health effects, and related information
- information about exposure limits, and whether OSHA, the International Agency for Research on Cancer, or the National Toxicology Program considers the chemical a carcinogen
- the primary routes of entry
- any generally applicable precautions for safe handling and use that are known to the preparer of the MSDS, including appropriate hygienic practices, protective measures during repair and maintenance of contaminated equipment, and procedures for cleanup of spills or leaks
- any generally applicable control measures that are known to the MSDS preparer, such as appropriate engineering controls, work practices, or PPE
- emergency and first-aid procedures
- the date of the MSDS preparation and identification of the party responsible for the MSDS

No blank spaces are permitted. When information is not available or is not applicable, spaces should be marked appropriately.

Chemical identities

Each MSDS must be written in English and contain the identity used on the label as follows:

- If the hazardous chemical is a single substance, its chemical and common name(s)
- If the hazardous chemical is a mixture that has been tested as a whole to determine its hazards, the chemical and common name(s) of the ingredients that contribute to these known hazards, and the common name(s) of the mixture itself

- If the hazardous chemical is a mixture that has not been tested as a whole, the chemical and common name(s) of all ingredients that have been determined to be health hazards and that compose at least 1% of the composition must be listed

However, chemicals identified as carcinogens must be listed if the concentration is 0.1% or greater. The chemical and common name(s) of all ingredients that have been determined to be health hazards and that comprise less than 1% (0.1% for carcinogens) of the mixture also must be listed if there is evidence that the ingredient(s) could be released from the mixture in concentrations that would exceed an established OSHA PELs or ACGIH TLV or could present a health hazard to employees. In addition, the chemical and common names of all ingredients that have been determined to present a physical hazard when present in the mixture must be listed.

Hazard determination

Chemical manufacturers and importers are required to evaluate chemicals they produce or import to determine whether they are hazardous. Employers are not required to evaluate chemicals unless they choose not to rely on the evaluation performed by the manufacturer or importer.

In making a hazard determination, available scientific evidence must be considered. For health hazards, evidence that is statistically significant and that is based on at least one positive study is considered sufficient to establish a hazard, if the results meet OSHA's hazard definitions.

Hazard determination of mixtures

Mixtures of chemicals also are subject to the hazard determination requirements. If a mixture as a whole has been tested for adverse health effects, those results should be used to make the health hazard determination. If such testing has not been done, the mixture must be assumed to present the same health hazards as any constituent chemical that comprises 1% or more of the mixture.

If a constituent chemical is 0.1% or more and is a carcinogen, the mixture must be considered carcinogenic. If a mixture component represents less than 1% but might result in workplace exposures that exceed OSHA PELs, the ACGIH TLV, or other harm to workers, this must be reported.

Chemicals that must be considered hazardous

Chemicals that should be treated as hazardous under the standard include those so listed in the following source:

- Air contaminants standard, Subpart Z, Toxic and Hazardous Substances, OSHA Threshold Limit Values for Chemical Substances and Physical Agents (current edition), published by the ACGIH

Carcinogen identification

A chemical must be considered to be a carcinogen or possible carcinogen for hazard communication purposes if so listed in the following sources:

- Annual Report on Carcinogens (latest edition), NTP
- The International Agency for Research on Cancer (IARC) Monographs (latest editions)
- Air contaminants standard, Subpart Z, Toxic and Hazardous Substances

In addition, the Registry of Toxic Effects of Chemical Substances published by NIOSH also indicates whether a chemical has been found by NTP or IARC to be a potential carcinogen.

Chemicals commonly used in laboratories and listed as carcinogens include ethylene oxide and formaldehyde.

Carcinogen label and MSDS requirements

The existence of positive human evidence on carcinogenicity always requires carcinogen warnings on the label of a hazardous substance, according to OSHA's hazard communication compliance directive.

There may be instances in which a carcinogen warning may be required for a chemical that is not listed by IARC or NTP but for which multiple animal studies indicate carcinogenicity. Such cases must be reviewed by the OSHA regional administrator and coordinated by the director of compliance and health standards programs.

Hearing/noise exposure (1910.95)

at a glance

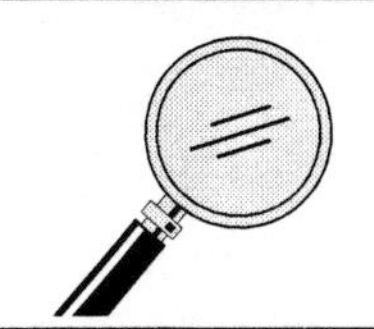

OSHA's noise standard regulates exposure levels through engineering controls (enclosing noisy equipment), PPE, and administrative controls (limiting duration of work).

Occupational hearing loss generally comes from damage to the inner ear due to excess noise exposure. Exposure to excessive noise over extended periods of time overstimulates and damages sensory mechanisms in the inner ear, which results in permanent hearing loss. Hearing loss also may be caused by damage to inner ear mechanisms from a sudden, very loud noise, such as an explosion. Temporary hearing loss can occur when the sensory mechanisms are not damaged but simply overstimulated and able to recover with time.

Excess noise is detrimental not only because it causes hearing loss but because it also can cause stress-related problems such as high blood pressure, muscle tension, headaches, decline in job performance, and depression. Excessive noise may create accidents and injuries if the noise makes it difficult for employees to hear warnings or instructions.

Employees should be able to hear coworkers speaking in a normal voice at arm's length; if someone consistently needs others to speak up so that he or she can hear them, the person should be tested for hearing loss. Employers and employees should be alert to other signs of hearing loss as well, such as tinnitus (a ringing in the ears) and difficulty in hearing that persists for a few hours after leaving a noisy area.

OSHA states that whenever noise exposure exceeds permissible levels, the levels must be reduced with feasible administrative controls (limiting duration of exposure) or engineering controls (enclosing noisy equipment). If such controls fail or are not feasible, PPE and hearing protectors must be provided to employees at no cost. Workers must be informed of the effects of noise on hearing; the purpose, fitting, and use of hearing protectors; and the purpose and procedures of audiometric testing.

Hearing conservation program

OSHA's hearing-protection standard (29 CFR 1910.95) requires employers to administer a continuing hearing conservation program whenever employee noise exposures equal or exceed an eight-hour TWA of 85 dBA. The hearing conservation program includes monitoring, audiometric testing, employee notification, personal protection, and training.

Monitoring

When any employee's noise exposure equals or exceeds the eight-hour TWA of 85 dBA, the employer must develop and implement a monitoring program. Monitoring should identify employees who need to be included in the program and enable employers to make the proper selection of hearing protectors. All continuous intermittent and impulsive sound levels from 80 dBA to 130 dBA must be integrated into the noise measurements. Monitoring has to be repeated whenever a change in production, process, equipment, or controls increases noise to an extent that may expose employees to unacceptable levels.

Employers must notify each employee exposed at or above an eight-hour TWA of 85 dBA of the results of monitoring.

Audiometric testing

The employer also must establish and maintain an audiometric testing program and make it available, at no cost, to all employees whose exposure equals or exceeds an eight-hour TWA of 85 dBA. Testing must be performed by a certified professional or qualified technician.

Hearing protectors

Hearing protectors must be available to all workers exposed at or above 85 dBA. Employers must provide the hearing protectors at no cost to employees and replace them when necessary.

Employees must be provided with and use hearing protection if they are exposed to a dBA of 90 or above or are exposed to an eight-hour TWA of 85 dBA or greater. Employees who have not yet had a baseline audiogram or have experienced an STS must also use hearing protection. An STS is a change in hearing threshold relative to the baseline audiogram of an average of 10 dB or more at 2,000, 3,000, and 4,000 hertz in either ear.

Employees should decide, with the help of a person trained in fitting protectors, which size and type of protector is most suitable.

The protector selected should be comfortable to wear and offer sufficient attenuation to prevent hearing loss. Employees must be shown how to use and care for their protectors and must be supervised to ensure that they continue to wear them correctly.

Hearing protectors must provide adequate attenuation for each employee's work environment. The employer must reevaluate the suitability of the employee's present protector whenever there is a change in working conditions that may cause the hearing protector to be inadequate. If workplace noise levels increase, employees must be given more effective protectors.

According to the OSHA Technical Manual, when the TWA exposure is less than 100 dB, hearing protectors may be used in lieu of engineering controls if certain conditions are met.

The protector must reduce employee exposures to a maximum of 90 dB, or to 85 dB when an STS has occurred.

Training

Workers who understand the reasons for the hearing conservation program's requirements will be better motivated to participate actively in the program and to cooperate by wearing protectors and taking audiometric tests.

A training program must be developed for all employees exposed to TWAs of 85 dBA and above. Training must be repeated annually and must include the

- effects of noise on hearing
- purpose, advantages, disadvantages, and attenuation of various types of hearing protectors, as well as information on selection, fitting, use, and care
- purpose and procedures of audiometric testing

Training does not have to be accomplished in one session. The program may be structured in any format, and different parts may be conducted by different individuals.

Monitoring and measuring noise

OSHA's hearing conservation amendment, 29 CFR 1910.95(c), requires employers to monitor noise exposure in a manner that will accurately identify employees who are exposed at or above 85 dBA, as measured on the eight-hour TWA. The exposure measurement must include all noise within a range of 80–130 dBA. The requirement is performance-oriented and allows employers to choose the monitoring method that best suits each individual situation.

Employees are entitled to observe monitoring procedures and, in addition, they must be notified of the results of exposure monitoring. The method used to notify employees is left to the employer's discretion.

Employers must remonitor workers' exposures whenever changes in exposures are sufficient to require new hearing protectors or cause employees who were previously not included in the program (because they were not exposed to an eight-hour TWA of 85 dBA) to be included in the program.

Within six months of an employee's first exposure to noise at or above a TWA of 85 dB, a valid baseline audiogram should be taken against which subsequent audiograms can be compared.

Instruments used to monitor employee exposures must be calibrated to ensure that the measurements are accurate. Calibration procedures are unique to specific instruments; employers should follow the manufacturer's instructions to determine when and how extensively to calibrate.

Noise exposure measurement records must be retained for two years. Audiometric test records must be retained for the duration of the affected worker's employment. Records should be made available upon request to employees, their designated representatives, former employees, and the assistant secretary of labor.

Audiometric testing program

The audiometric testing program includes baseline audiograms, annual audiograms, training, and follow-up procedures. The program should indicate whether hearing loss is being prevented by the employer's hearing conversation program. Audiometric testing must be made available at no cost to all employees who have average exposure levels of 85 dB.

Both professionals and trained technicians may conduct audiometric testing. In addition to administering audiometric tests, the tester also is responsible for ensuring that the tests are conducted in an appropriate test environment, that the audiometer works properly, and that the audiograms are reviewed for STS. An STS is a change in hearing threshold relative to the baseline audiogram of an average of 10 dB more at 2,000, 3,000, and 4,000 hertz in either ear.

If a technician conducts the tests, he or she either must be certified by the Council of Accreditation in Occupational Hearing Conservation or have demonstrated competence in conducting tests.

Audiograms

Employers are required to make both baseline and annual audiograms. The baseline audiogram is the reference audiogram against which future audiograms are compared. Baseline audiograms must be provided within six months of an employee's first exposure at or above a TWA of 85 dBA.

Where employers are using mobile test vans to obtain audiograms, baseline audiograms must be completed within one year after an employee's first exposure. Employees who are exposed at or above 85 dB for more than six months before having a baseline audiogram must be provided with and wear hearing protectors from the time they are exposed over the initial six months until they receive baseline audiograms.

Employees must experience at least 14 hours without exposure to workplace noise before a baseline audiogram is taken. Hearing protectors may be used in order to comply with this requirement. Employers also must notify employees to avoid high levels of nonoccupational noise during the 14 hours preceding the test.

Employees who are exposed to noise at levels at and above 85 dB must be tested annually within one year of the baseline test. This is done so that changes in hearing acuity can be detected and protective follow-up measures can be initiated before hearing loss progresses.

Audiogram evaluation

Annual audiograms must be compared routinely to baseline audiograms to determine whether the audiogram is accurate and to determine whether the employee has lost hearing ability (that is, whether an STS has occurred).

If an STS is identified, employees must be fitted or refitted with adequate hearing protectors, shown how to use them, and required to wear them. In addition, employees must be notified within 21 days from the time their audiometric test results show an STS.

Some employees with an STS may need to be referred for further testing if the professional determines that their test results are questionable or if they have an ear problem of a medical nature caused or aggravated by wearing hearing protectors. If the suspected medical problem is not thought to be related to wearing protectors, employees merely must be informed that they should see a physician.

If subsequent audiometric tests show that the STS identified on a previous audiogram is not persistent, employees whose exposures are less than a TWA of 90 dBA may discontinue the wearing of hearing protectors.

Where a baseline audiogram is revised due to an STS or an improvement in hearing, the employer must retain the original audiogram.

Audiometric test requirements

Audiometric examinations must be conducted with test frequencies including a minimum 500, 1,000, 2,000, 3,000, 4,000, and 6,000 hertz. Tests for each frequency must be taken separately for each ear.

Audiometric tests must be conducted as specified by the noise standard. Audiometers must be used, maintained, and calibrated according to the noise standard's specifications.

Medical referral

The American Academy of Otolaryngology—Head and Neck Surgery Foundation, Inc. recommends that medical referrals be kept to a minimum because they are both costly and time-consuming. However, in cases of doubt, it is better to refer someone who did not need to be referred than not to refer someone who should have been referred. Physicians should be consulted in cases of doubt.

The academy's audiologic criteria for referral to a specialist for threshold shifts seen on periodic audiograms should be distinguished from criteria for threshold shifts used to trigger in-house action, such as refitting of hearing protectors, by the hearing conservation program.

The academy recommends that, for baseline audiograms, referrals be made when the average hearing level at 500, 1,000, 2,000, and 3,000 hertz is greater than 25 dB in either ear.

Referrals also should be made when the difference in average hearing level between the better and poorer ear is greater than 15 dB at 500, 1,000, and 2,000 hertz, or when it is greater than 30 dB at 3,000, 4,000, and 6,000 hertz.

Evaluation table

Table 1 at the end of this chapter will assist in evaluation of the noise levels in the workplace. When employees are subjected to sound levels that exceed those listed in the table, feasible administrative or engineering controls must be used. If these controls do not work, PPE must be provided.

When the daily noise exposure is composed of two or more periods of noise exposure of different levels, their combined effect should be considered, rather than the individual effect of each. If the sum of C1/T1 + C2/T2 + . . . Cn/Tn exceeds unity, then the mixed exposure should be considered to exceed the limit value. Cn indicates the total time of exposure at a specified noise level in hours, and Tn indicates the total time of exposure permitted at that level.

Exposure to impulsive or impact noise should not exceed 140 dB peak sound pressure level.

A noise survey performed by adequately equipped and trained personnel should be made before engineering and administrative controls are put into effect or a hearing conservation program is established.

Table 1

Permissible noise exposures

Duration per day: Hours	Sound level dBA Slow response
8	90
6	92
4	95
3	97
2	100
1.5	102
1	105
0.5	110
0.25 or less	115

Laboratory standards (1910.1450)

at a glance

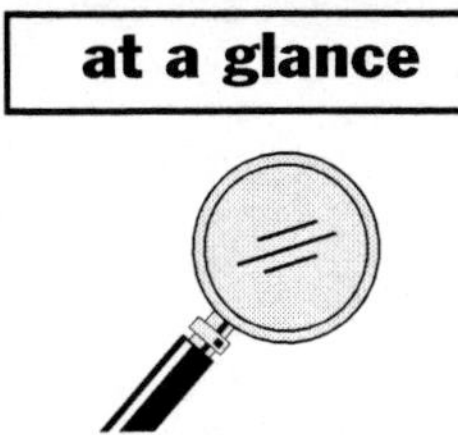

OSHA's hazardous chemicals in laboratories standard protects laboratory workers from occupational exposure to hazardous chemicals in the workplace. The standard covers hazard-identification labels and MSDSs. It also refers to other standards, including respiratory protection, fire prevention and protection, chemical spills, and recordkeeping.

The OSHA laboratory standard applies to facilities that fall within the agency's definition of laboratory use and laboratory scale.

Laboratory use means the handling or use of hazardous chemicals in which all of the following conditions are met:

- The size and frequency of chemical manipulations are those of a typical laboratory (they are on a "laboratory scale")
- More than one chemical or chemical procedure is used
- The procedures used are not part of a production process, and they do not simulate a production process in any way
- Protective laboratory practices are in effect, and equipment is available and in common use

Laboratory scale refers to the relatively small quantities of hazardous chemicals used in the workplace, including work in which the following occurs:

- The containers used for reactions, transfers, and other handling of substances are designed to be used easily and safely by one person.
- The workplace does not produce commercial quantities of materials. The lab may produce materials for use outside the lab (e.g., in another part of the facility).

OSHA makes no exception based on the size of the laboratory. For example, even clinical laboratories operated part-time in medical offices by nurses or technicians must comply with the standard if they use hazardous substances.

Hazardous substances covered

The laboratory standard covers all chemicals defined as hazardous under the OSHA hazard communication standard (29 CFR 1910.1200). This means that any chemical for which the hazard communication standard requires manufacturers to provide an MSDS must be addressed under the laboratory standard.

PELs

For laboratory uses of OSHA-regulated substances, employers must ensure that lab workers are not exposed to those substances in excess of the PELs. PELs are established under OSHA's standards for toxic and hazardous substances, 29 CFR 1910, Subpart Z.

Additionally, more stringent precautions must be taken under the laboratory standard when certain "select" carcinogens, reproductive-hazardous substances, or acutely hazardous substances are being handled. The standard defines a select carcinogen as any substance that is

- regulated by OSHA as a carcinogen
- included as a known carcinogen in the National Toxicology Program's Annual Report on Carcinogens
- in Group 1 of the International Agency for Research on Cancer's latest monograph

Laboratory employers also are required to determine when special precautions should be taken for chemicals that are suspected carcinogens or target organ toxins.

Monitoring

The employer must measure the employee's exposure to any substance regulated by an OSHA standard that requires monitoring if there is reason to believe that exposure levels for that substance routinely exceed the action level or PEL. If that initial monitoring discloses employee exposure over the action level or PEL, the employer must comply immediately with the exposure-monitoring provisions of the relevant standard until the exposure level is brought within permissible limits. The employer must notify employees of the results of the monitoring within 15 working days after they are known. The notification must be in writing and may be given to employees individually or posted in an appropriate place where employees will see it.

CHP

Employers are required by the standard to have a written CHP. The CHP is to be implemented for the laboratory in general and must automatically cover any hazardous chemical present. The CHP must be reviewed at least annually, updated as necessary, and be readily available for employees or their representatives and for OSHA upon request. Although certain elements must be addressed by the CHP, the particular details are left to the employer's discretion.

Required plan elements

Specific elements are required in the CHP to ensure employee protection from hazardous-chemical exposures. The plan must include the following:

- SOPs relevant to safety and health that will be followed when lab work involves the use of hazardous chemicals

- Criteria that the employer will use to determine and carry out control measures—including engineering controls, the use of PPE (e.g., respirators, appropriate gloves), and hygiene practices—to reduce employee exposure

- Specific measures for ensuring that fume hoods and other protective equipment are functioning properly

- Provisions for employee information and training

- Operations, procedures, or activities that require prior approval by the employer

- Provisions for medical consultation and examination, when appropriate

- Provisions for additional employee protection for working with extremely hazardous substances

- Designation of a CHO who should be experienced and qualified to provide technical assistance in the development and administration of the CHP

SOPs

SOPs ensure that the laboratory follows written work practices and policies that protect employees from chemical hazards. Such procedures explain general safety precautions, including the following:

- Using safety glasses, general housekeeping practices, and restrictions on eating and drinking
- Correct responses to emergencies
- Proper methods of cleaning up hazardous-chemical spills and disposing of such substances

Criteria for reducing exposure

The CHP must list criteria for deciding when to institute measures to control exposure. Such measures include engineering controls, use of PPE, and hygiene practices.

The laboratory standard recommends that the criteria address several issues, including the following:

- The chemicals used and the degree of hazard they present

- The potential for exposure from the procedures used

- The ability of the engineering controls, administrative practices, and protective equipment to control exposure
- How frequently the lab performs the operations that may expose workers to hazardous chemicals
- The presence of open vessels
- The proximity of other workers who may not be adequately protected
- The predictability of the operation's outcome
- Past experience with the operation or substances

Fume hoods and other protective equipment

Fume hoods and ventilation systems are the chief mechanical means for controlling exposure to hazardous chemicals. The laboratory standard requires that all hoods and other protective equipment function properly at all times, and that the laboratory employer demonstrate how proper performance is ensured.

The CHP should specify the "face velocities" (the rate at which air is drawn into the hood from the laboratory area immediately surrounding it) needed in the laboratory, based on chemicals used and operations performed. The plan should describe the inspection and maintenance program used to keep hoods functioning at their most effective rate.

Proper hood-use techniques to achieve maximum exposure reduction also should be addressed. For example, exposure will be significantly less if substances are poured or otherwise handled at least six inches inside the hood. Also, workers should not put their heads inside a hood while hazardous materials are being released. Storage of chemicals in hoods should be prohibited.

The CHP should show how to maintain other protective equipment, such as respirators and glove boxes. All laboratories must have emergency respirators, which must meet respiratory-protection provisions under OSHA's standard for respiratory protection (29 CFR 1910.134).

Employee information and training

The standard requires employers to provide information and training in both the physical and health hazards associated with the chemicals in the employees' work areas. This training and information must be provided at the time of an employee's initial assignment and prior to assignments that involve new hazardous chemicals or new exposure situations. The required training does not necessarily involve training for each specific chemical that the employee will use, but it may be directed to classes or groups of hazardous chemicals.

The CHP should explain why certain employees are trained, when they are trained, and how often they are retrained. The plan also should describe the training program, list each hazardous substance for which training is provided, and explain how employees are trained to handle each substance.

Information requirements

Information to be communicated and made available to employees includes the following:

- Contents of the standard and its appendices.

- The employer's CHP.

- The PELs for OSHA-regulated substances used in the work area as well as for other hazardous chemicals.

- Signs and symptoms associated with exposures to hazardous chemicals used in the laboratory.

- The availability of reference materials on the hazards, safe handling, storage, and disposal of hazardous chemicals. Reference material includes but is not limited to MSDSs that may be available from chemical suppliers.

Training requirements

Employee training must include the following:

- How the employer and employees can detect the presence or release of a hazardous chemical in the work area. This should include training on environmental and medical monitoring, use of monitoring devices, and the appearance and odor of hazardous chemicals being released. Employees should be trained to recognize any release alarm or warning system used in the lab.

- The physical and health hazards of the chemicals in the work area, including fire and explosions, how a chemical enters the body, and effects of exposure. Where large numbers of chemicals are used, separate training sessions on each chemical or chemical category may be necessary.

- How employees can protect themselves from the hazards of the chemicals with which they work. This should include information about safe work practices, emergency procedures, and using PPE that the employer provides. Protection by engineering controls also should be explained.

- The details of the lab's CHP, including an explanation of the labeling system, MSDSs, and how employees can obtain and use hazard information.

Prior employer approval

Certain chemicals and operations are so hazardous that they should be supervised more carefully than others. The CHP should require workers to obtain their supervisor's approval before they start conducting operations that involve acutely toxic substances, highly volatile material, or embryotoxins.

Uses of certain chemicals should be reviewed at regular intervals and each time procedures change. The CHP should give supervisors authority to impose additional precautions for operations that require their approval.

Prior approval should be required for any operation that

- the lab has not conducted previously
- involves using new chemicals and/or chemicals the lab has not used previously, whether in a new operation or in an operation the lab already performs
- may yield a compound with unknown byproducts or intermediates

The plan should identify which chemicals or classes of chemicals and which operations require prior approval. It also should specify who has the authority to approve operations and under what circumstances written approval is required.

Medical consultation and examinations

The standard requires that employers provide all employees who work with hazardous chemicals the opportunity to receive, at no cost to the employees, appropriate medical attention, as necessary. Employees must have the opportunity for medical examinations whenever they exhibit signs or symptoms associated with exposure to a hazardous chemical.

Employees also must have the opportunity for a medical consultation whenever there is an event in the work area, such as a spill, leak, explosion, or other occurrence that could result in a significant risk of chemical exposure. The medical consultation is provided for the purpose of determining the need for a medical examination.

Where exposure monitoring reveals an exposure level routinely above the action level or the PEL for an OSHA-regulated substance, the medical surveillance requirements of the particular standard that governs that substance must be established for the affected laboratory employee.

All medical examinations and consultations must be performed by, or under the direct supervision of, a licensed physician; be provided at a reasonable time and place; and be provided at no cost to employees.

The employer must provide the examining physician with the identity of the hazardous chemicals to which the employees have been exposed, a description of the conditions under which the exposure occurred, and a description of the signs and symptoms of the exposure.

The employer must obtain from the examining physician a written opinion that includes a statement that the employee has been informed of the results of the examination and any medical condition that might require further treatment.

Additional protective precautions

The standard requires that the CHP include the following provisions to protect employees who work with particularly hazardous substances:

- Establishment of a designated area—that is, an area that may be used only for work with select carcinogens, reproductive toxins, or acutely toxic substances

- Use of containment devices, such as fume hoods or glove boxes

- Procedures for the safe removal of contaminated wastes

- Decontamination procedures

The "designated area" is identified by posting a warning sign to let employees know that they are in the presence of hazardous chemicals or operations. The chemicals or class of chemicals that are used in the area, and the kinds of hazards they pose, should be specified.

CHO

Every laboratory must have a CHO to develop and administer the CHP. If appropriate, a chemical-hygiene committee should be appointed as well.

Under the laboratory standard, the CHO must be "qualified by experience or training to carry out these responsibilities." Potential CHO candidates could include a health and safety officer, laboratory supervisor, or any other individual with appropriate experience or training.

The CHO, facility administrators, and lab employees should develop the facility's laboratory policies and practices. The CHO should do the following:

- Monitor procurement, use, and disposal of hazardous chemicals used in the laboratory
- Maintain an auditing program
- Help project directors develop adequate facilities and precautions in their CHPs or standard operating procedures
- Be thoroughly versed in laboratory-operations law

Hazard identification

Employers must ensure that labels on incoming containers of hazardous chemicals are not removed or defaced and must maintain the MSDSs that come with those chemicals. Hazard identification requirements fall under both the laboratory standard and OSHA's hazard communication standard (29 CFR 1910.1200). To avoid any confusion between the two standards, OSHA makes the following clarifications:

- If a chemical substance whose composition is known is produced in the laboratory for the laboratory's exclusive use, OSHA's laboratory standard requires that available hazard information be provided to employees who may be exposed to the substance. MSDSs and label preparations as required under the hazard communication standard do not apply.

- Laboratory employers that produce a chemical byproduct whose composition is unknown must make the assumption that the substance is hazardous and must require that it be handled according to the employer's CHP.

- If a chemical is produced in the laboratory and shipped to another user outside the laboratory, the employer has become a manufacturer with respect to the substance produced and therefore is subject to all relevant provisions of the hazard communication standard, including requirements for the development of MSDSs and labeling.

Respirators

The employer must provide, free of charge, appropriate respirators for employees when it is necessary to use the devices in order to maintain exposure below PELs.

When there is no PEL designated by OSHA for a hazardous substance used in a laboratory, the agency's standard for respiratory protection must be followed (29 CFR 1910.134).

Recordkeeping

The laboratory standard requires that the employer provide and maintain for each employee an accurate record of any measurements taken to monitor employee exposures and any medical consultation and examination records required by OSHA (29 CFR 1910.1020). Specifically, the provisions require that employers keep these records for the duration of employment plus 30 years.

Generally, employers must keep any record created in connection with the laboratory standard. These records include the following:

- Medical records, such as a copy of a doctor's report on an examination a lab employee had to undergo to meet requirements of the standard. Such records also might include medical or employment histories, laboratory test results, medical opinions or progress notes, first-aid reports, descriptions of treatments and prescriptions, or an account of an employee's medical complaints.

- Exposure records, including background data on environmental monitoring and measuring, which only must be kept for one year. The sampling plan and its results, a description of the analytical and mathematical methods used, and a summary of other background data needed to interpret the results must be kept for 30 years after the employee retires. Other exposure records include results of environmental or biological monitoring for the presence of hazardous substances.

- MSDSs. Although chemical-inventory records are not required to be kept, some record must be kept of the identity of substances used, how they were used, and when they were used.

- Inspection dates and findings for respirators that are maintained in the lab for emergency use.

Current employees, former employees, and employees assigned or transferred to work where they will be exposed to toxic substances must be allowed to inspect their records. Access also must be allowed to employees' designated representatives—any person or organization to whom the employee or the employee's estate gives written authorization.

Collective-bargaining agents are considered designated representatives and do not need the employee's authorization to see the records.

Healthcare-facility laboratories

General laboratory areas in healthcare facilities present both health and safety hazards. Pathology and autopsy areas can be a source of biological hazards. Infectious diseases can be transmitted to employees through poor work practices such as eating, drinking, and smoking in the laboratory and pipetting by mouth. A statement of facility policy prohibiting these activities should be provided to each employee, be prominently posted, and be strictly enforced.

Management must provide safe and healthful working conditions. Employees are responsible for following facility policy and using the health and safety controls provided by management. Managers should also ensure that the lab's EC policies are specifically tailored to the lab, and not simply dictated by what the rest of the facility does.

Work-practice guidelines

Important considerations and specific work-practice guidelines that should be included in a CHP designed for laboratory employees include the following:

- Do not eat, drink, or smoke in the lab. Food and beverages should not be stored in refrigerators or anywhere in the lab.
- Never pipette by mouth.
- Wear coats or aprons while in the lab, and remove them when leaving the area.
- Wear appropriate goggles or face shields when doing work that could involve accidental splashes to the face or eyes.
- Obtain emergency care for all injuries, no matter how slight. Be aware of any break in the skin where chemicals or biological agents could enter. Make sure these agents don't come in contact with the broken skin.
- Know the proper disposal method for all chemicals used in the laboratory, as well as for radioactive wastes, specimens, cultures, and analytical chemicals.
- Use separate containers for the disposal of glass, syringes, and needles. Cuts, bruises, and puncture wounds may be caused by improper disposal of these items.

- Keep flammable materials in approved safety containers. Keep no more than one day's supply in the work area outside of an approved storage cabinet. Refrigerators used for the storage of flammables must be of the explosion-proof type.

- Use an exhaust hood when working with toxic, flammable, or volatile materials.

PPE

Appropriate safety goggles and/or face shields must be provided, and their use must be enforced in areas or during operations where chemicals or other hazardous substances can be accidentally splashed into the eyes.

Eyewash facilities and safety showers must be immediately available if acids or caustics are used in the laboratory, and employees should be trained in the proper use of these facilities. The areas around these facilities must be kept clear at all times. The facilities should be tested regularly to ensure proper working conditions.

A chemical cartridge respirator for use with acid gases and organic vapors should be readily available for use during cleanup of spills. The respirator should be stored immediately outside the laboratory.

Fire extinguishing equipment

A dry chemical (A:B:C) or carbon dioxide (B:C) extinguisher should be present in any clinical lab.

Because the amount of flammable liquids and chemicals vary between labs, it is important to evaluate each specific hazard before determining the proper selection and placement of fire extinguishers. In some cases the value or importance of delicate equipment in a lab often dictates the use of the special and more expensive fire extinguishers containing clean halogenated agents or alternatives.

NFPA 99, *Standard for Health Care Facilities*, requires labs to have extinguishers suitable for the particular hazards of a lab (paragraph 10-5.3).

All extinguishers must be properly mounted and maintained, and the areas around the equipment must be kept clear at all times.

Facilities should train all employees in the proper use of fire extinguishers if they are expected to use them during a fire. Lab employees must also be ready to deal with a situation in which someone's clothing catches fire.

Laboratory hoods and ventilation

Exhaust-ventilation hoods are required in laboratories where toxic chemicals and biological materials are handled. The Industrial Ventilation Manual published by the ACGIH provides information on hood design for specific applications.

An exhaust-ventilation hood should be designed to capture a contaminant at its source. There is no hood that has universal application. Slotted-side draft hoods along the back of a lab bench may be adequate for open bench tops. Small canopy hoods may be sufficient to capture the contaminant released by a piece of analytical test equipment. Completely enclosed hoods (ventilated glove-box type) should be used for highly toxic chemicals or highly infectious specimens.

The ventilation rates of all hoods should be measured, the data recorded, and the measurements kept near the hoods for future reference. The entire ventilation system should be routinely monitored (monthly) to check its efficiency. It is suggested that a pressure-sensing gauge be installed where the hood enters the duct work to measure the "hood static pressure." This gauge can be visually monitored daily to determine whether the system is working properly. This gauge can be red-lined to indicate acceptable operating conditions.

Chemical fume hoods should be designed for an average face velocity of 100 fpm, or 150 fpm if the hood is used for toxic work (substances with threshold limit values less than 10 ppm or 0.1 milligram per cubic meter).

Laboratory equipment

All electrical equipment (including radios, fans, etc.) must be grounded effectively. The disconnects for all equipment must be properly marked, and the areas around the breaker boxes must be kept clear.

Wiring and connections on all electrical equipment should be checked regularly, as rotating, moving, and vibrating equipment may wear the insulation or put tension on the terminal screws.

Compressed-gas cylinders must be secured and kept upright, and the valve-protection caps must be fastened when not in use. Compressed-gas hoses, fittings, and gauges must be kept in good condition and checked periodically for leaks.

Working areas that have been contaminated with infectious biological cultures should be cleaned with an effective disinfectant.

Chemicals and biologicals

Laboratory work requires the use of many different chemicals and agents. Chemicals used often vary from week to week, depending on the nature of the work being done.

The following are recommendations for controlling employee exposures to health and safety hazards that may be present in the laboratory.

Chemical-list compilation

Compile a list of the common agents used in each laboratory. This list should include the following:

- Organic compounds, such as organic solvents (e.g., xylene, formaldehyde, acetone)
- Inorganic compounds, such as heavy metals (e.g., mercury)
- Physical hazards (e.g., ultraviolet radiation, ultrasonic devices)
- Biological hazards (e.g., virus [hepatitis and HIV] and bacteria [tuberculosis])

Hazard communication

Educate employees who are potentially exposed to the hazards of the substances with which they work on how to recognize symptoms of exposure and the effects of overexposure.

Exposure monitoring

Monitor employees' exposures to ensure that airborne concentrations of the contaminants are below the allowable limits. For information about techniques for air sampling, contact the NIOSH industrial hygienist in your area or a state or local industrial-hygiene office.

Collect biological samples to monitor employees' exposures to toxic substances (e.g., mercury in the blood, hippuric acid in the urine for toluene exposure, enzyme activity levels, etc.).

Storage, handling, and disposal procedures

Establish a procedure for the proper storage, handling, and disposal of all chemicals. Establish a procedure to ensure that biological safety cabinets are decontaminated routinely and certified annually.

Chemical-spill procedures

Establish a detailed chemical-spill procedure. Appropriate neutralizing substances should be easily accessible for emergency use.

Check floors and benches for accumulations of spilled mercury.

Post names and telephone numbers of persons to be notified in emergency situations. This is particularly important in large research-laboratory facilities that perform experimental work.

Lasers (guidance)

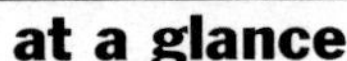

at a glance

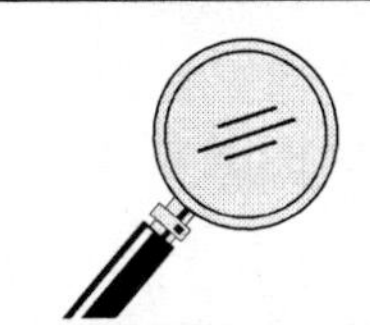

OSHA outlines laser classification and sets control measures to minimize laser hazards. The PPE (1910.132) and eye and face protection (1910.133) standards apply. Safety programs should include an LSO, SOPs, controlled access areas, and PELs.

OSHA has issued a guidance on laser hazards for federal and state compliance officials to use when conducting workplace inspections. The guidelines outline laser classification and set control measures that should be used to minimize laser hazards.

The following four basic categories of controls are useful in laser environments:

- Administrative and procedural
- Engineering
- PPE
- Special controls

The OSHA guidelines are based on voluntary safety recommendations issued by ANSI. The guidelines instruct federal and state inspectors to check for safety-program components such as

- an appointed LSO
- SOPs
- operator training and qualifications
- maximum PEL
- controlled-access areas

Employers also are required to post hazard warning signs in areas where lasers are in use or are undergoing service.

Lasers in laboratories

LASER is an acronym that stands for Light Amplification by Stimulated Emission of Radiation. A laser is a concentrated, high-power beam of light. Although lasers can be quite powerful, the most significant characteristic of a laser is not its total power but the power per unit area (i.e., the focus of the laser's total power on a very small spot).

Lasers used in laboratories usually are referred to according to the lasing media contained in the tube.

Lasers are categorized from Class I, which generally includes the least hazardous devices, to Class IV, which includes those that have the greatest potential to cause injury.

Potential hazards

Laser systems can present serious occupational hazards if not managed and used properly. Direct or reflected laser beams can cause irreversible damage to the eyes and skin of exposed workers. Permanent blindness is one potential hazard. Lasers also may cause tissue damage.

Ultraviolet energy may result in radiation carcinogenesis. Additionally, evidence is accruing that smoke produced during laser use (i.e., laser plume) may contain toxic chemicals and viable biological contaminants that pose other health risks.

Lasers present safety risks as well. The intense heat can cause fires when flammable items are in close proximity to the beam. The high-voltage electricity required to power some lasers presents a risk of electrical shock.

Federal safety requirements

OSHA does not have a standard for laser use in laboratories. Citations for unsafe working conditions related to the use of lasers in laboratories may be issued under the general duty clause of the Occupational Safety and Health Act, which requires employers to maintain a safe and healthful workplace, or under the standard for PPE, which requires employers to provide appropriate PPE where needed.

Laser manufacturers are subject to general performance requirements issued by the Center for Devices and Radiological Health, which is part of the FDA. The federal laser-product performance standard (21 CFR 1040) impacts worker safety to the extent that it requires manufacturers of lasers to report on performance features, such as protective housings, warning labels, safety interlocks, emission indicators, and scanning-beam safeguards.

ANSI standards

ANSI has two standards on laser use that have special pertinence to laboratory facilities:

ANSI standard Z136.1 applies to laser use in multiple industries. The standard describes the concept of the NHZ, establishes maximum PELs, describes the laser-classification scheme, specifies recommended control measures, outlines suggested medical-surveillance practices, and specifies personnel-training requirements.

ANSI standard Z136.3 provides more specific guidance for healthcare employers. This standard provides recommendations on the safe use of lasers for diagnostic and therapeutic purposes and covers occupational health risks related to air contaminants (e.g., laser plume) and electrical and fire hazards. Control measures specific to healthcare applications—such as safety audits, foot pedals, output calibration, and quality control—are given additional coverage.

Types of laser-induced tissue damage

Laser radiation can cause serious, irreversible damage to human eyes and skin. The degree of damage that a given laser can inflict usually is commensurate with factors such as the intensity of heat generated by the laser, the length of exposure time, the size of the area irradiated, and the extent of local vascular flow.

The most common cause of laser-induced tissue damage is heat. Thermal damage or burns are associated with lasers operating at exposure times greater than 10 microseconds and in the wavelength region from the near ultraviolet to the far infrared (0.315–103 micrometers (µm)). Tissue damage also may be caused by thermally induced acoustic waves following exposures to submicrosecond laser exposures.

Other damage mechanisms have been demonstrated for specific wavelength ranges and/or exposure times. Photochemical reactions (i.e., where tissue/cell chemistry is disrupted) are the principal cause of tissue damage following exposures to either actinic ultraviolet radiation (200–315 nm) for any exposure time or "short wave" visible radiation (400–550 nm) when exposures are greater than 10 seconds. Skin damage such as hyperpigmentation and erythema can be caused by UV-A (315–400 nm). In addition to thermal injury caused by ultraviolet energy, there is the possibility of radiation carcinogenesis from UV-B (280–315 nm) either directly on DNA or from effects on potentially carcinogenic intracellular viruses.

Basic safety-program requirements

A comprehensive laser-safety program is key to protecting workers from laser-related accidents and injuries. According to ANSI safety standards and the OSHA inspection guidelines, laser-safety programs should have as a foundation

- a qualified LSO who is assigned to be the responsible leader and coordinator of the program
- a written SOP for identifying laser hazards and implementing appropriate controls

Other control measures that should be part of the program include

- administrative and equipment controls
- procedural controls
- laser controlled areas
- maintenance and service controls
- PPE
- warning signs and labels

Role of the LSO

The LSO should have the authority to monitor and enforce the control of laser hazards and to affect the knowledgeable evaluation and control of laser hazards.

The LSO should administer the overall laser-safety program where the duties include but are not limited to

- confirming the classification of lasers
- conducting the NHZ evaluation
- ensuring that the proper control measures are in place and approving substitute controls
- approving SOPs
- recommending/approving eyewear and other protective equipment
- specifying appropriate signs and labels
- approving overall facility controls
- providing the proper laser-safety training, as needed
- conducting medical surveillance
- designating the laser and incidental-personnel categories

Hazard evaluation

A hazard evaluation is a tool used to determine the safety-control measures required for the lasers used in a given location.

According to the ANSI standard, the following four aspects of the healthcare laser system influence the total hazard evaluation and thereby influence selection of the control measures to be applied:

- The capability of the radiant energy of the laser system to injure personnel or the patient's body area other than the intended treatment sites
- The environment in which the laser system is used
- The personnel who may use, or be exposed to, laser radiation
- The non-emission hazard associated with the laser system

SOP

An SOP is required for all Class IV lasers and laser systems and is recommended for Class IIIB lasers, according to OSHA.

The key to a successful SOP is involvement of the individuals that operate, maintain, and monitor/service the equipment. Topics that may be covered in the written SOP include preoperative, intraoperative, and postoperative safety precautions, maintenance/service schedules and procedures, and fire prevention and emergency action plans.

Administrative and procedural controls

Administrative and procedural controls that should be addressed in the safety program include the following:

- **Alignment procedures**—Alignment tasks spur a large portion of the laser eye accidents that occur each year. Therefore, alignment procedures should be undertaken only with extreme caution. A written SOP is recommended for all recurring alignment tasks.
- **Limitations on spectators**—Persons unnecessary to the laser operation should be kept away. Those who do enter the laser area should wear appropriate protective eyewear and receive safety instruction.

- **Protective equipment**—Protective equipment for laser safety may include eye protection in the form of goggles or spectacles, clothing, barriers, and other devices designed for laser protection. OSHA's PPE standard (29 CFR 1910.132-.140) may apply in some cases.

- **Laser barriers and protective curtains**—Special barriers, designed to withstand laser beams, are available for the purpose of area control. If used, such barriers should be placed at an appropriate distance and should be made of material that does not support combustion in the event of an exposure.

NHZ

In addition to laser classification, a laser's ability to injure personnel depends on its NHZ—the space within which the level of direct, reflected, or scattered radiation exceeds the MPE limits.

The LSO should determine the NHZ for all Class IV and Class IIIB lasers and use this information to determine the region where control measures are required. Persons outside of the NHZ are exposed below the MPE limit and are considered to be in a "safe" location.

The following laser characteristics should be used to determine the NHZ:

- Power or energy output
- Beam diameter
- Beam divergence
- Pulse-repetition frequency
- Wavelength
- Beam path, including reflections
- Beam profile
- Maximum anticipated exposure duration

Operator qualifications/credentials

The most important aspect of a laser-safety program may be the skill and safety awareness possessed by the laser operator. Generally, responsibility for determining whether an individual is capable and qualified to operate a laser safely lies with the laboratory facility.

OSHA inspectors may consider factors such as the laser operator's level of expertise, understanding of potential hazards, and knowledge of safety practices when conducting workplace inspections.

General safety procedures

Engineering controls normally are designed and built into laser equipment to provide for safety. In most cases, they will be included on the equipment as part of the performance requirements mandated by the FDA's federal laser-product performance standards, which regulate the manufacturers of commercial laser products.

An important general safety precaution is that the LSO be notified of the purchase of any laser, according to OSHA. Notification should include information such as the laser's classification, media, output power, wavelength, beam size at aperture, and potential or designated users.

Other general precautions include the following:

- Shiny or glossy objects should not be placed into the laser beam, unless specifically designed for use with that equipment. Use of anodized or other nonreflecting instruments generally is recommended.

- Eye protection should be provided whenever engineering controls are insufficient to eliminate the possibility of any hazardous eye exposure. Such devices should be designed for protection against radiation from a specific laser system and should be labeled with optical-density values and wavelengths for which protection is afforded.

- Skin protection is best achieved through engineering controls. However, skin covers or "sun screens" may be recommended for use with ultraviolet lasers. Most gloves provide some protection against laser radiation. Flame-resistant clothing may be considered for use with Class IV lasers.

Environment

To determine whether the control measures are adequate, it is important to consider the environment in which the laser is used. When analyzing laser environment, at a minimum, the following must be considered:

- Number of lasers or laser systems
- Degree of isolation
- Probability of the presence of uninformed, unprotected transient personnel
- Permanence of beam paths
- Permanence of specularly reflecting objects in or near the beam path
- The use of optics (e.g., lenses, microscopes, optical fibers)

Engineering controls

Lasers generally come equipped for use with engineering controls devised by the manufacturer. Such controls may include the following:

- **Protective housing**—An enclosure around the laser that either limits access to the laser beam or keeps radiation at or below the applicable MPE level is required. A protective housing is required for all classes of lasers, except at the beam aperture.

- **Protective-housing interlock**—Interlocks that cause beam termination or reduction of the beam to MPE levels should be provided on all panels intended to be opened during operation and maintenance of all Class IIIA, Class IIIB, and Class IV lasers. The interlocks are typically electrically connected to a beam shutter; when a panel is displaced or removed, the shutters close and eliminate the possibility of hazardous exposures.

- **Master-switch control**—All Class IV lasers require a master-switch control. The switch can be operated by a key or computer code. When disabled (key or code removed), the laser cannot be operated. Only authorized system operators are to be permitted access to the key or code.

- **Optical-viewing system**—Interlocks, filters, or attenuators are to be incorporated in conjunction with beam shutters when optical-viewing systems such as telescopes, microscopes, viewing ports, or screens are used to view the beam or beam-reflection area. For example, an electrical interlock could prevent laser-system operation when a beam shutter is removed from the optical-system-viewing path. Such optical-filter interlocks are required for all but Class I lasers.

- **Beam stop or attenuator**—Class IV lasers require a permanently attached beam stop or attenuator that can reduce the output emission to a level at or below the appropriate MPE level when the laser system is on "standby."

- **Laser-activation-warning system**—An audible tone or bell and/or visual warning (such as a flashing light) is mandatory for Class IV lasers. Such warning devices are to be activated upon system startup and are to be uniquely identified with the laser operation. Verbal "countdown" commands are an acceptable audible warning and should be a part of the SOP.

- **Service-access panels**—Protective housing that is to be removed only by service personnel to permit direct access to an embedded Class IIIB or Class IV laser should either have an interlock or require that a tool is used in the removal process. If an interlock is used and is defeatable, a warning label indicating this fact is required on the housing near the interlock.

- **Remote interlock connector**—Class IV lasers are provided with a remote interlock connector to allow electrical connections to an emergency master disconnect ("panic button") interlock or to room, door, or flucture interlocks. When open-circuited, the interlock should cause the accessible laser radiation to be maintained below the appropriate MPE level.

PPE

In cases where controls such as beam enclosure are not sufficient to eliminate laser-exposure hazards, PPE may be required. Generally, this translates into the use of laser-safety eyewear and, in some cases, protective clothing. However, respirators, hearing protection, laser-barrier devices, curtains, and filtered or covered viewing windows also may be required to afford adequate protection, according to the OSHA inspection guidelines.

Nonbeam-laser hazards should be considered in the selection of PPE, including eyewear. These hazards may include laser-induced fumes and vapors, flammable or toxic chemicals and materials, electrical power supplies, and noise.

Protective eyewear

Eye-protection devices designed to protect against radiation from a specific laser system must be used when engineering controls are inadequate to eliminate the possibility of potentially hazardous eye exposure. Appropriate protective eyewear should be worn by all persons within the NHZ whenever operational conditions may result in a potential eye hazard. This includes laboratory personnel, patients, and visitors or family members who are allowed to be present. According to OSHA, use of protective eyewear is mandatory for personnel in the controlled area where Class IV lasers are used.

The eyewear should reduce potential ocular exposure below MPE limits and, when worn, should cover the cornea, conjunctiva, and other ocular tissue. Protective eyewear should be fabricated of plastic or glass absorption filters appropriate for the laser. All laser-protective eyewear should be clearly labeled with optical-density values and wavelengths for which protection is afforded. The manufacturer of the eyewear should supply this information to the purchaser along with other pertinent safety data. Color-coding or other distinctive identification is recommended by ANSI for multiple-laser environments.

All personnel using Class IIIB and Class IV lasers should be provided information necessary to make the correct and optimum choice of laser-protective eyewear. This means, in general, that they need a more complete understanding of such topics as

- the specific wavelength(s) of the laser emission.
- exposure time of anticipated or "worst-case" exposure.
- the output parameters of the laser in use. This includes the average laser power or pulse energy, pulse lengths, and pulse repetition characteristics.

- worst-case ocular-exposure levels.
- the "safe" exposure criteria of maximum permissible exposure for each laser.
- in some cases, aspects of the viewing condition (e.g., point source or extended source).
- reflection factors from targets at the laser wavelength.
- optical density of eyewear at laser-output wavelength.
- visible-light-transmission requirements.
- radiant exposure or irradiance at which laser-safety-eyewear damage occurs.
- need for prescription glasses.
- comfort and fit.
- degradation of absorbing media.
- strength of materials (resistance to shock).
- need for peripheral vision.
- specifications of the protective devices commercially available.

It is recommended that other controls be employed rather than relying solely on the use of protective eyewear because many accidents have occurred when eyewear was available but not worn. There are many reasons cited for this problem, but the most common is that laser-protective eyewear is often dark, is uncomfortable to wear, and limits vision.

Laser barriers and protective curtains

In some cases, area control of the laser beam can be accomplished using special barriers designed to withstand direct and/or diffusely scattered beams.

The barrier should be labeled with a Barrier Threshold Limit (BTL) (i.e., beam penetration through the barrier after a specified exposure time, typically 60 seconds). The barrier should be located at an appropriate distance from the laser source so that the BTL is not exceeded in the worst-case exposure scenario. An analysis usually is required to establish the recommended barrier type and installation distances for a given laser. Important in the design is the flammability of the barrier. It is essential that the barrier not support combustion or be consumed by flames following an exposure.

Protective viewing windows

According to OSHA, all viewing portals, optics, windows, or display screens included as a part of the laser or laser installation should incorporate a means to lessen the intensity of the laser radiation transmitted through to levels below the appropriate MPE levels. The filtration chosen should be based upon the level of laser radiation that would occur at the window in a typical worst-case condition.

Protective clothing

In cases where personnel may be exposed to levels of radiation that clearly exceed the MPE for the skin, particularly in the ultraviolet, the LSO should recommend or approve the use of protective clothing. Where personnel may be subject to chronic skin exposure from scattered ultraviolet radiation, skin protection should be provided even at levels below the MPE for skin.

Consideration also should be given to the use of fire-resistant clothing when using Class IV lasers. Skin protection is best achieved through engineering controls. However, if the potential exists for damaging skin exposure, particularly for ultraviolet lasers (200–400 nm), then skin covers and/or sunscreen creams are recommended. For hand protection, most gloves will provide some protection against laser radiation. Tightly woven fabrics and opaque gloves provide the best protection. A laboratory jacket or coat can provide protection for the arms. For Class IV lasers, consideration should be given to flame-resistant materials.

Laundry/housekeeping

(various standards, including 1910.264 [laundry machinery and operations], 1910.1030 [bloodborne pathogens], 1910.1200 [hazard communication], 1910.22 [walking-working surfaces], and 1910.141 [general environmental controls])

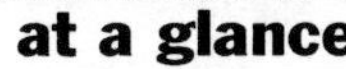

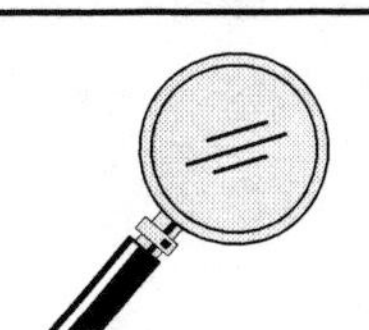

The laundry standard applies to moving parts of equipment used in laundries and to specific conditions related to the industry. The standard does not apply to dry-cleaning operations. The standards protect workers from infection, hazards inherent in the work, and mechanical injuries.

OSHA's laundry machinery and operations standard, which makes special reference to the point of operation of laundry machines, requires

- every washing machine, drying tumbler, and shaker in a laundry to be set up so that the door of the machine can be held open while the machine is loaded and unloaded.

- all steam pipes within seven feet of the floor or working platform, and those that workers might touch, to be insulated, covered with heat-resistant material, or otherwise guarded.

- proper protection to be provided to prevent injury or damage caused by fluid escaping from relief or safety valves, if vented to the atmosphere.

- markers or other workers who handle soiled clothes to be warned against touching the eyes, mouth, or any part of the body on which the skin has been broken by a scratch or abrasion. They also must be warned not to touch or eat food until their hands have been thoroughly washed.

- employees to be trained, through bulletins, printed rules, and verbal instruction, to recognize the hazards of their work and to carry out safe work practices.

- that no safeguard or safety appliance on any machinery be removed except to repair or adjust the equipment. Any safety device removed must be replaced immediately upon completion of repairs or adjustments.

OSHA's lockout/tagout standard applies to the servicing and maintenance of machines in which the unexpected energization or startup of a machine or release of stored energy could cause injury to employees (29 CFR 1910.147). The standard requires the control of hazardous-energy sources by means of lockout/tagout procedures to disable machinery or equipment during maintenance and/or servicing.

Bloodborne pathogens

It is the employer's responsibility to determine which employees are at risk of exposure to bloodborne pathogens and therefore are entitled to coverage under OSHA's bloodborne-pathogens standard (29 CFR 1910.1030). Occupations covered under the standard include personnel in hospital laundries or commercial laundries that service healthcare or public-safety institutions where occupational exposure to blood or OPIM occurs.

The bloodborne-pathogens standard requires the following:

- Contaminated laundry must be handled as little as possible. It must be bagged or put in containers at the location where it was used, but it cannot be sorted or rinsed in that location.
- Bags or containers in which the laundry is placed and transported must be labeled or color-coded to permit all employees to recognize the containers as having contaminated contents.
- When contaminated laundry is wet, it must be placed and transported in bags or containers that prevent soak-through or leakage to the exterior.
- If UP are used for handling all soiled laundry, the employer may use an alternative color or label for the bags/containers, as long as all employees are trained to recognize them.

Appropriate PPE, such as gloves, must be worn by employees who have contact with contaminated laundry. It is the employer's responsibility to ensure that workers comply with this requirement.

In addition, employers are responsible for cleaning, laundering, and disposing of PPE at no cost to employees. The equipment must be repaired and replaced as needed to maintain its effectiveness. This, too, must be at no cost to employees.

Garments penetrated by blood or OPIM must be removed immediately or as soon as feasible. All PPE must be removed before leaving the work area.

Off-site shipment violations

If contaminated laundry is shipped to another facility for cleaning, the following constitute violations of the bloodborne-pathogens standard:

- The contaminated laundry is not shipped in a properly labeled bag or in a red bag
- The contaminated laundry is shipped with an improper label
- The contaminated laundry is shipped in a bag color-coded for in-house use

Hazard communication

Laundry operations also are regulated by OSHA's hazard-communication standard (29 CFR 1910.1200), which addresses employees' exposure to hazardous chemicals. The standard requires that employees be

- informed of the requirements of the standard, any operations in their work area where hazardous chemicals are present, and the location and availability of the written hazard-communication program. This includes the required list of hazardous chemicals and MSDSs.

- informed of procedures for determining the presence of hazardous chemicals, specific hazards of specific chemicals, and the protective measures the employer has developed for employees to follow.

- trained in how to read and interpret information on labels and MSDSs and how to obtain and use the available hazard information.

Laundry workers may come into contact with solvents and other flammable and combustible liquids. Employers should establish procedures for handling such hazardous materials, including good housekeeping practices, proper ventilation, and the use of PPE.

Asbestos

OSHA's general industry standard for asbestos (29 CFR 1910.1001) requires that clothing contaminated with asbestos fibers not be taken out of the change room, except by employees authorized to do so for the purpose of laundering, maintenance, or disposal. Contaminated work clothing must be placed and stored in closed containers to prevent the dispersion of asbestos. The containers must be labeled appropriately.

Employers may not allow employees to remove asbestos from protective clothing or equipment by shaking or blowing. Laundering contaminated clothing must be done in a manner that does not release airborne asbestos fibers above the permissible exposure limits. Workers laundering the clothing must be informed of this requirement.

Formaldehyde

Protective equipment and clothing contaminated with formaldehyde must be cleaned or laundered before its reuse, as required under OSHA's formaldehyde standard (29 CFR 1910.1048). The standard also requires containers for contaminated clothing and equipment and storage areas to have appropriate labels and signs.

Only persons trained to recognize the hazards of formaldehyde may be allowed to remove the contaminated material from the storage area for cleaning, laundering, or disposal. Any person who launders, cleans, or repairs such clothing or equipment must be informed of formaldehyde's potentially harmful effects and of procedures to safely handle the clothing and equipment.

Training requirements

OSHA's laundry machinery and operating rules require employees to be properly instructed as to the hazards of their work and to be instructed in safe practices. For training purposes, employers may use bulletins, printed rules, and verbal instructions.

The bloodborne-pathogens standard has specific training requirements and a set of specific precautions that must be followed by workers who may come into contact with blood or OPIM.

The hazard-communication standard requires employers to provide employees with information and training on hazardous chemicals in their work area at the time of their initial assignment and whenever a new hazard is introduced into their work area.

Health and safety program

NIOSH issued guidelines to reduce the incidence of injury and disease among healthcare workers. The following elements should be included in a health and safety program for laundry workers:

- Floors should be kept as dry as possible, and wet floors should be labeled. Nonskid mats or flooring should be provided in wet areas, and workers should wear nonskid boots or shoes.

- Laundry should be handled as if hazards were present because puncture wounds and cuts can result from needles, knives, and blades that are folded into soiled linens.

- Soiled linens should be handled as little as possible with minimum agitation to prevent contamination of the air. All soiled linens should be bagged with impervious, color-coded bags at the site where they are used, and materials contaminated with potentially infective agents, cytotoxic drugs, or radionuclides should be clearly labeled and handled with special care. To protect workers from unnecessary contact, a barrier should separate soiled-linen areas from the rest of the laundry area.

- The high temperatures and excessive humidity in some laundry areas may be impossible to control with engineering devices alone, especially during the summer months. Administrative controls may be necessary, and persons working in excessively hot environments can be rotated to other jobs or shifts.

- Workers should be aware of the symptoms of heat stress and the need for water consumption and more frequent breaks.

- Workers who sort and wash contaminated linens should wear proper protective clothing and respirators.

- Workers should be trained in the proper techniques for lifting and material handling.

- Laundry personnel should be instructed to wash their hands thoroughly before eating, drinking, and smoking; before and after using toilet facilities; and before going home.

- Workers who handle and sort soiled linen in the laundry department should be included in the laboratory immunization program.

- The wrapping on steam lines should be maintained adequately to protect workers from burns.

- Proper precautions should be taken when handling soaps and detergents (e.g., gloves should be worn, substitutes should be used for known sensitizers, etc.).

Eliminating unsafe practices

NIOSH suggests that employers take the following steps to help reduce unsafe acts and practices in the workplace:

- Impress upon workers the need for constant safety awareness—even during automatically controlled operations

- Be sure that all employees know when and how to use appropriate PPE
- Develop and maintain checkpoints to be observed as a part of standard and emergency procedures during each shift
- Post appropriate warning signs and operating procedures
- Instruct employees in the use of portable fire extinguishers
- Have at least one person trained in first aid on each shift
- Be sure that employees who are authorized to use motorized equipment are thoroughly instructed in its operation and potential hazards
- Develop good housekeeping awareness to reduce accidents and to promote employee pride in the workplace environment
- Instruct employees in safe-lifting practices
- Never permit employees to use solvents as hand cleansers because they remove the natural oils from the skin and many may be absorbed through the skin, which could cause liver and kidney damage

The CDC recommends the following infection-control measures:

- Immunizations for vaccine-preventable diseases
- Isolation precautions to prevent exposures to infectious agents
- Management of personnel exposures to infected persons, including postexposure prophylaxis
- Work restrictions for exposed or infected personnel

Housekeeping standards

General housekeeping requirements are included in OSHA's standard for walking-working surfaces (29 CFR 1910.22). The standard requires

- all places of employment, including passageways, storerooms, and service rooms, to be kept clean and orderly and in a sanitary condition.
- the floor of every workroom to be kept clean and, wherever possible, dry. Where wet processes are used, drainage must be maintained, and false floors, platforms, mats, or other dry standing places should be provided where practicable.
- to facilitate cleaning, every floor, working place, and passageway to be kept free from protruding nails, splinters, holes, or loose boards.
- where mechanical handling equipment is used, sufficient safe clearances to be allowed for aisles, at loading docks, through doorways, and wherever turns or passage must be made.
- aisles and passageways to be kept clear and in good repair, with no obstruction across or in aisles that could create a hazard. Permanent aisles and passageways must be appropriately marked.
- covers and/or guardrails to be provided to protect workers from the hazards of open pits, tanks, vats, ditches, etc.

The bloodborne-pathogens standard also applies to housekeeping operations. The standard requires that the work site be maintained in a clean and sanitary condition. Employers are required to implement an appropriate written schedule for cleaning and for methods of decontamination. In addition, the standard requires that

- all equipment and working surfaces be cleaned and disinfected after contact with blood or OPIM

- protective coverings such as plastic wrap, aluminum foil, or imperviously backed absorbent paper used to cover equipment and environmental surfaces be removed and replaced as soon as possible after they become contaminated or at the end of the work shift if they have become contaminated during the shift

- all bins, pails, cans, and similar receptacles intended for reuse be inspected and decontaminated regularly, or cleaned and decontaminated immediately if there is visible contamination

The hazard-communication standard requires employers to inform housekeeping employees of the potential health hazards associated with exposure to chemicals used or stored in the workplace. The standard requires a written hazard-communication plan, warning labels on containers, distribution of MSDSs, and employee-training programs.

Workplace hazards

Housekeeping workers are potentially exposed to many health and safety hazards found in the laboratory environment. NIOSH recommends that housekeeping workers receive periodic instruction to keep them aware of the specific hazards in the laboratory.

The guidelines address the following hazards often encountered by housekeeping workers:

- Medical waste presents a potential hazard for housekeeping and environmental-services workers responsible for cleaning and waste collection within healthcare facilities. Normally, housekeeping workers do not generate the waste but may be responsible for waste segregation, handling, storage, and on-site treatment. They risk exposure to hepatitis and other diseases from hypodermic needles that have not been properly discarded.

- Sprains and strains are common problems for housekeepers. Housekeeping workers often experience back problems due to lifting and setting down objects and using scrubbing machines, brooms, and mops.

- Soaps and detergents may cause dermatitis or sensitization reactions. Workers should be trained to use these materials properly and should be provided with appropriate protective gloves. Effective cleaning solutions that do not cause dermatitis or sensitization should be substituted when possible. Sensitized workers should be transferred to other duties if necessary.

- Solvents, such as methyl ethyl ketone, acetone, and Stoddard solvent, often are used to clean grease from equipment and may have several cleaning applications throughout the laboratory facility. Workers should be instructed in their proper use to prevent both fire hazards and exposures that could lead to illness. Many solvents remove the natural fats and oils from the skin and, when absorbed through the skin, can cause respiratory effects. Appropriate PPE should be worn by workers who come into contact with solvents.

- Cleaners used throughout the laboratory may contain acids or caustics that can cause burns. Workers who use these solutions should wear proper protective clothing such as rubber gloves, rubber or plastic aprons, and eye protection.

- Disinfectants are often used in laboratories. Because many disinfectants can produce skin rashes and dermatitis, PPE for the skin and eyes is required.

- Bacteria and viruses, to which housekeeping personnel are frequently exposed, may present a potential health hazard. Such personnel should follow instructions issued by the infection-control department for reporting infections. Workers also should take appropriate measures to limit further contagions from patients by practicing UP for handling blood and body fluids.

Health and safety program

NIOSH recommends the following guidelines for a health and safety program for housekeeping workers:

- Workers should be trained in proper material-handling techniques.

- Workers should be instructed to wash their hands thoroughly before eating, drinking, and smoking; before and after using toilet facilities; after removing contaminated work gloves; and before going home.

- Workers should be aware that other persons may not have followed proper procedures for disposing of needles, knives, and glassware. All refuse should be handled as if hazardous items were present.

- Workers should seek help either from other persons or from mechanical devices when lifting or moving equipment or furniture that is heavy or awkward.

- Workers may be injured as a result of improper use and poor maintenance of ladders, step stools, and elevated platforms. To reduce the frequency of falls, workers should not stand on the top two steps of a ladder and should not substitute chairs, boxes, or other items for a ladder.

- All electrical appliances, such as vacuums and polishers, should have grounded connections.

- Service carts should be equipped with large, wide wheels to make them easier to push.

- The slippery areas on floors that are being scrubbed or polished should be identified with signs or roped-off areas.

Sanitation requirements

Workplace sanitation requirements are included in OSHA's standard for general environmental controls (29 CFR 1910.141). In addition to general housekeeping requirements, the standard requires that

- safe drinking water be provided in all places of employment. The use of a common drinking cup is forbidden.

- receptacles for waste food be covered and kept in a clean and sanitary condition.

- separate toilet facilities be provided for each sex. If only one person at a time uses a toilet room and the door can be locked from the inside, separate facilities are not required.

- one toilet and one lavatory be provided for approximately every 15 employees.
- each lavatory have hot and cold or tepid running water, hand soap, and individual hand towels or warm-air blowers.
- beverages or food not be stored or consumed in a toilet room or in any area exposed to toxic materials.
- employees working with toxic substances wash and, where necessary, change from contaminated clothing before eating, drinking, or smoking.
- for wet processes, drainage be maintained and dry standing places be provided, where practicable, or appropriate waterproof foot gear must be provided.

Lead (1926.62 [construction work] and 1910.1025 [general industry])

at a glance

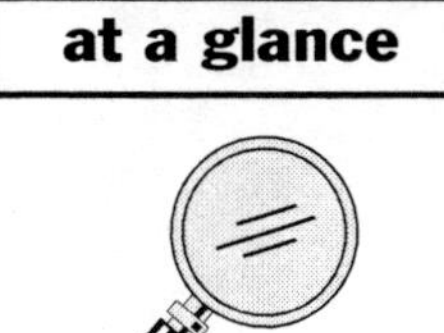

The lead standard covers exposure levels, monitoring exposure, compliance programs, respiratory protection, PPE, training, and recordkeeping. Remodeling, painting, or lead-disturbing maintenance could trigger the standard.

The OSHA lead standard for general industry (29 CFR 1910.1025) applies to all occupational exposure to lead, except for exposure associated with the construction industry or agricultural operations. Building-maintenance activities, which include making or keeping a structure, fixture, or foundation in proper condition in a routine, scheduled, or anticipated fashion, are covered by the general industry standard.

PELs

OSHA's PEL is 50 micrograms of lead per cubic meter of air ($\mu g/m^3$) as an eight-hour TWA. For employees exposed to lead for more than eight hours in any work day, the PEL equals 400 $\mu g/m^3$ divided by the number of hours worked in that day. When respirators are used to supplement engineering and work-practice controls and all respiratory requirements have been met, employee exposure may be considered to be at the level provided by the protection factor of the respirator for the periods the respirator is worn.

The action level of employee exposure, without regard to the use of respirators, is set at 30 $\mu g/m^3$ as an eight-hour TWA. Exposures exceeding the action level trigger certain monitoring and other protective requirements.

Monitoring requirements

The general industry lead standard has provisions for initial determination of exposure and necessary periodic monitoring. Under these requirements, employee exposure is that which could occur if the employee were not using a respirator. Employers must use a method of monitoring and analysis with an accuracy (to a confidence level of 95%) of not less than +/- 20% for airborne concentrations of lead equal to or greater than the action level of 30 $\mu g/m^3$.

Initial monitoring

Employers must collect full-shift (for at least seven continuous hours) personal samples, including at least one sample for each shift for each job classification in each work area. The samples must represent the employee's regular, daily exposure to lead. The employer must make initial determinations of exposure based on monitoring results and any of the following:

- Any information, observations, or calculations that would indicate employee exposure to lead
- Any previous measurements of airborne lead
- Any employee complaints, kept in their original state, of symptoms that may be attributable to lead

If the determination shows the possibility of any employee exposure at or above the action level, the employer must conduct monitoring representative of all employee exposure to lead in the workplace. Measurements made in the preceding 12 months may be used to satisfy this requirement if the sampling and analytical methods meet accuracy- and confidence-level requirements.

If a determination is made that no employees are exposed at or above the action level, the employer must make a written record of the determination.

Periodic monitoring

When initial determination reveals employee exposure to be at or above the action level but below the PEL, the employer must repeat the monitoring process at least every six months. The employer must continue the monitoring until two consecutive measurements, taken at least seven days apart, are below the action level.

If initial determination reveals employee exposure above the PEL, monitoring must be repeated quarterly. The employer must continue the monitoring until two consecutive measurements, taken at least seven days apart, are below the PEL. If the consecutive measurements are below the PEL but at or above the action level, six-month monitoring must continue until two consecutive readings fall below the action level.

Changes in production, process, control, or personnel that may result in increased lead exposure, or any expectation thereof, must warrant additional monitoring.

Employee notification

Employees must be notified in writing of their individual exposure-monitoring results within five working days after employer receipt of the results. If exposure, without regard to respirators, exceeds the permissible limit, the employer must include in the written notice a statement that the PEL was exceeded and a description of the corrective action taken or to be taken to reduce exposure to or below the limit.

Methods of compliance

If any employee is exposed to lead above the PEL for more than 30 days per year, the employer must implement engineering and work-practice controls (including administrative controls) to reduce and maintain employee exposure to lead, except to the extent that the employer can demonstrate that such controls are not feasible. If controls do not reduce exposure to or below the PEL, the employer must supplement them with respirators.

If all employees are exposed to lead above the PEL for 30 days or less per year, the employer must implement engineering controls to reduce exposure to 200 $\mu g/m^3$, and then may implement any combination of engineering, work-practice, and respiratory controls to further reduce and maintain employee exposure to lead to or below the PEL of 50 $\mu g/m^3$.

Written compliance program

Affected employers must create a written compliance program to reduce exposures to or below the PEL, and interim levels if applicable, solely by means of engineering and work-practice controls. Written plans must include at least the following:

- A description of each operation in which lead is emitted
- A description of the specific means used for compliance, including engineering plans and studies
- A report of the technology considered in meeting the PEL
- Air-monitoring data documenting the source of lead emissions
- A detailed schedule for implementation of the program, including documentation such as construction contracts, etc.
- A work-practice program
- An administrative-control schedule, if applicable
- Other relevant information

Written programs must be submitted upon request to OSHA, and must be available at the work-site for examination and copying by OSHA, any affected employee, or authorized employee representatives.

Mechanical ventilation

When ventilation is used to control exposure, measurements that demonstrate the effectiveness of the system to control exposure, such as capture velocity, duct velocity, or static pressure, must be made at least every three months. Measurements must be made within five days of any change in production, process, or control that might change employee exposure.

If air from exhaust ventilation is recirculated into the workplace, the employer must ensure that the system has a high-efficiency filter with a reliable back-up filter. The employer must maintain effective controls to monitor the concentration of lead in the return air and to bypass the recirculation system automatically if it fails.

Administrative controls

If administrative controls are used as a means of reducing employee exposure, the employer must implement a job-rotation schedule that identifies each affected employee, describes duration and exposure levels at each job or work station where each affected employee is located, and includes any other information useful in assessing the reliability of administrative controls.

Respiratory protection

OSHA's general industry standard for lead includes respiratory-protection provisions (29 CFR 1910.1025[f]) for employees who use respirators for lead-related activities. Employers must provide the respirators and ensure that they are used during

- periods necessary to install and implement engineering or work-practice controls
- work operations for which engineering and work-practice controls are not sufficient to reduce exposures to or below the PEL
- periods when an employee requests a respirator

Respirator program

Where respiratory protection is required, the employer must implement a respirator program in accordance with applicable requirements of OSHA's respiratory-protection standard (29 CFR 1910.134).

If an employee has breathing difficulty during fit testing or respirator use, the employer must provide a medical examination to determine whether the employee can use a respirator while performing the required duty.

Respirator selection

When certain airborne concentrations of lead or conditions of use are encountered in the work environment, the employer must select and provide the appropriate respirator as specified in Table 1 at the end of this chapter. The employer must provide a tight-fitting PAPR instead of the respirator specified in Table 1 when an employee chooses to use this type of respirator, as long as the PAPR provides adequate protection.

Respirator fit testing

Under the respiratory-protection standard (29 CFR 1910.134[f]), before an employee may be required to use any respirator with a negative- or positive-pressure tight-fitting facepiece, the employee must be fit tested with the same make, model, style, and size of respirator to be used. Such employees must pass an appropriate qualitative or quantitative fit test prior to initial use of the respirator, whenever a different respirator facepiece is used, and at least annually thereafter. Additional fit tests may be required as necessary.

Additional requirements

The respiratory-protection standard also includes requirements for respirator use, maintenance, and care; breathing-air quality and use; identification of filters, cartridges, and canisters; employee training and information; respirator-program evaluation; employee medical evaluation; and recordkeeping.

Protective clothing and equipment

For any employee exposed to lead above the PEL, the employer must both provide free of charge and ensure the use of appropriate protective clothing and equipment such as coveralls or similar full-body work clothing; gloves, hats, and shoes or disposable shoe coverlets; and face shields, vented goggles, or other appropriate protective equipment.

The employer must provide the protective clothing and equipment in a clean and dry condition at least weekly, and daily to employees whose exposure levels are over 200 $\mu g/m^3$ as an eight-hour TWA. Employers must repair or replace required clothing and equipment as needed to maintain effectiveness.

Employers must ensure that all protective clothing is removed at a shift's end, in designated changing rooms. The employer must ensure that contaminated clothing in need of cleaning, laundering, or disposal is placed in a closed container in the changing room. Employers must prohibit blowing, shaking, or any other means of removing lead from protective clothing or equipment, if that means could disperse lead into the air.

The employer must label the clothing containers as follows:

CAUTION: CLOTHING CONTAMINATED WITH LEAD. DO NOT REMOVE DUST BY BLOWING OR SHAKING. DISPOSE OF LEAD-CONTAMINATED WASH WATER IN ACCORDANCE WITH APPLICABLE LOCAL, STATE, OR FEDERAL REGULATIONS.

Employers must inform in writing any person who cleans or launders protective clothing or equipment of the potentially harmful effects of lead exposure.

Housekeeping

All surfaces must be maintained as free as practical of lead accumulation. Floors and other surfaces where lead accumulates may not be cleaned using compressed air. Shoveling, dry or wet sweeping, and brushing may be used only where vacuuming or other equally effective methods have been tried and found ineffective. Vacuums should be used and emptied in a manner that minimizes reentry of lead into the workplace.

Hygiene facilities and practices

Employers must ensure that in areas where lead is above the PEL, food or beverage is not present or consumed, tobacco products are not present or used, and cosmetics are not applied.

Change rooms

Employers must provide clean change rooms for employees who work in areas where airborne-lead exposure is above the PEL. The change rooms must be equipped with separate storage facilities for protective work clothing and equipment and street clothes, to prevent cross-contamination.

Showers

The employer must ensure that employees shower at a shift's end if they work in areas where airborne exposure to lead is above the PEL. The employer must provide the shower facility. Employers must prohibit employees who exit the workplace from wearing any clothing or equipment worn during work.

Lunchrooms

Employers must provide lunchroom facilities for employees who work in areas where airborne exposure to lead is above the PEL. The employer must ensure that the facilities have a temperature-controlled, positive-pressure, filtered air supply, and are readily accessible to employees. Employers must ensure that employees who work in areas where airborne lead is above the PEL wash their hands before eating, drinking, smoking, or applying cosmetics. Employers must prohibit employees from entering the lunchroom with protective clothing or equipment unless surface lead dust has been removed by vacuuming, downdraft booth, or other cleaning method.

Medical surveillance

The employer must institute a medical-surveillance program for all employees who are or may be exposed above the action level for more than 30 days per year. All medical examinations and procedures must be performed by or under the supervision of a licensed physician, at no cost to the employee and at a reasonable time and place. Provisions of the medical surveillance program include the following:

- Biological monitoring in the form of blood sampling and analysis for lead and zinc protoporphyrin levels must be made available to each employee at least every six months. For employees whose last blood sampling and analysis indicated a blood lead level at or above 40 μg/100 g of whole blood, sampling and analysis must be made available every two months. Within five working days after the receipt of the results, the employer must notify in writing each employee whose blood lead level exceeds 40 μg/100g.

- Medical examinations and consultations must be made available to each covered employee. This must be at least annually for any employee whose blood-sampling test conducted at any time during the preceding 12 months indicated a blood lead level at or above 40 μg/100 g. Content of the examinations must be determined by a physician and include various provisions.

- A multiple-physician review mechanism must be offered to an employee if the employer selects the initial physician who conducts any medical examination or consultation provided to the employee. The employee may designate a second physician to review the initial physician's findings and to conduct further examinations and tests if necessary. The employer must promptly notify an employee of the right to a second medical opinion. The employee has 15 days from either receipt of the notice of the right to a second opinion or receipt of the initial physician's findings, whichever is later, to both inform the employer of intention to seek a second opinion and to take steps to make an appointment.

- Written medical opinions must be made available by the employer to an employee for each examining or consulting physician.

Medical-removal protection

Employees whose blood lead level is at or above 60 μg/100 g of whole blood or whose average blood level from three consecutive tests is at or above 50 μg/100 g must be removed from work. The employee need not be removed if the last blood test indicated a level at or below

40 µg/100 g. In addition, employees who receive a final medical determination resulting in a medical finding, determination, or opinion that the employee has a detected medical condition that places the employee at increased risk also will be removed. An employer may remove an employee from lead exposure when not required to do so but then must provide medical-removal benefits.

Removal benefits

Upon the employee's return from removal, the employer must return the employee to his or her former job status. Employers must not return an employee to work until appropriate medical determination has occurred.

The employer must provide up to 18 months of medical-removal protection benefits to the removed employees on each occasion of removal. The employer must maintain the earnings, seniority, and all other employment rights and benefits of an employee. The employer may require medical surveillance of the employee as a condition of these benefits.

Employers may credit against their obligation to the employee any earnings compensation resulting from workers' compensation claims, any earnings compensation from publicly or employer-funded compensation programs, and any income from employment with another employer made possible by virtue of the employee's removal.

For employees whose blood lead levels do not adequately decline in the 18-month period, the employer must do the following:

- Make available to the employee a medical examination to obtain a final medical determination

- Ensure that the final medical determination obtained indicates whether the employee may be returned to his or her former job status, and, if not, what steps should be taken to protect the employee's health

- Continue to provide medical protection benefits to the employee until either the employee is returned to former job status or a final medical determination is made that the employee is incapable of ever safely returning to his or her former job status

- Where a final medical determination allows the employer to return to work an employee with an otherwise unacceptable blood lead level, the employer must use a final medical determination to answer future removal questions and does not need to use the normal blood lead level criteria

Training

Where there is a potential exposure of airborne lead at any level, employers must inform employees of the contents of Appendices A and B of the OSHA general industry lead standard (29 CFR 1910.1025). The employer must institute a training program for and ensure the participation of all employees who are subject to exposure to lead at or above the action level or for whom the possibility of skin or eye irritation exists. Employees must be trained prior to initial job assignment, and the program must be repeated at least annually. The content of the training program should include

- the content of the OSHA general industry lead standard (29 CFR 1910.1025) and its appendices

- the specific nature of the operations that could result in exposure to lead above the action level

- the purpose, proper selection, fitting, use, and limitations of respirators

- the purpose and description of the medical-surveillance program and medical-removal protection program, with highlights about adverse health effects

- the engineering controls and work practices associated with the employee's job assignment

- the contents of any compliance plan in effect
- instructions to employees that chelating agents should not be used routinely to remove lead from their bodies and should not be used at all except under the direction of a licensed physician

The employer must make available to affected employees copies of the OSHA general industry lead standard (29 CFR 1910.1025), its appendices, and other materials pertaining to the OSHA. The employer must provide these and other training materials to OSHA upon request.

Signs

The employer must post in each work area where the PEL is exceeded signs that state the following:

WARNING

LEAD WORK AREA

POISON

NO SMOKING OR EATING

The signs must be illuminated and cleaned as necessary so that the legend is readily visible.

Observation of monitoring

Employers must provide affected employees or their designated representatives an opportunity to observe any monitoring of employee exposure to lead. Employers must supply the observer with respirators, protective clothing, or equipment when observers enter areas that require such protection. Observers are entitled to

- receive an explanation of the measurement procedures
- observe all steps related to the monitoring of lead performed at the place of exposure
- record the results obtained or receive copies of the results when returned by the laboratory

Table 1

Respiratory protection for lead aerosols

Airborne concentration of lead or condition of use	Required respirator[1]
Not in excess of 0.5 mg/m^3 (10 x PEL)	1. Half-mask air-purifying respirator equipped with high-efficiency filters[2,3]
Not in excess of 2.5 mg/m^3 (50 x PEL)	1. Full facepiece air-purifying respirator equipped with high-efficiency filters[3]
Not in excess of 50 mg/m^3 (1,000 x PEL)	1. Any PAPR with high-efficiency filters[3] 2. Half-mask supplied-air respirator operated in positive-pressure mode[2]
Not in excess of 100 mg/m^3 (2,000 x PEL)	1. Supplied-air respirators with full facepiece, hood, helmet, or suit operated in positive-pressure mode
Greater than 100 mg/m^3, unknown concentration, or firefighting	1. Full-facepiece SCBA operated in positive-pressure mode

Note:

1. Respirators specified for high concentrations can be used at lower concentrations of lead.
2. Full facepiece is required if the lead aerosols cause eye or skin irritation at the use concentrations.
3. A high-efficiency particulate filter means 99.97% efficient against 0.3 micron-sized particles.

Lockout/tagout (1910.147)

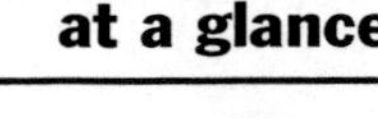

Whenever service or maintenance is performed on machines and equipment, OSHA requires that it be done with all equipment stopped and isolated from all sources of energy to minimize exposure to hazards from unexpected machine energizing.

The standard covers the servicing and maintenance of machines and equipment in which the unexpected energization or start-up of the machines or equipment, or release of stored energy, could cause injury to employees (29 CFR 1910.147[a]).

The standard does not cover

- construction, agriculture, and maritime employment
- installations under the exclusive control of electric utilities for the purpose of power generation, transmission, and distribution, including related equipment for communication or metering
- exposure to electrical hazards from work on, near, or with conductors or equipment in electric-utilization installations
- oil and gas well-drilling and servicing

The standard applies to the control of energy only during maintenance and/or servicing of machines and equipment. Normal production operations are not covered, unless

- an employee is required to remove or bypass a guard or other safety device
- an employee is required to place any part of his or her body into an area on a machine or piece of equipment where work is actually performed, such as the point of operation, or where a danger zone exists

The standard also does not apply to hot tap operations.

When other standards require lockout/tagout, they must be supplemented by the requirements of this standard.

Energy-control program

The employer must establish an energy-control program that includes written procedures for the control of potentially hazardous energy when employees are engaged in maintenance and/or servicing activities (29 CFR 1910.147[c]).

The program procedures must clearly outline the scope, purpose, authorization, rules, and techniques to be used for the control of hazardous energy and the methods of compliance, including

- a specific statement of the intended use of the procedures
- steps for shutting down, isolating, blocking, and securing machines or equipment to control hazardous energy
- steps for the placement, removal, and transfer of lockout or tagout devices and the responsibility for them
- requirements for testing a machine or equipment to determine and verify the effectiveness of lockout/tagout devices and other energy control measures used

The energy-control program also must include procedures for conducting periodic (at least annual) inspections of the program to ensure that it meets the standard's requirements.

Equipment isolation

The employer must ensure that before any employee performs any servicing or maintenance on a machine or equipment, the machine or equipment is isolated and rendered inoperative.

If an energy-isolating device is capable of being locked out, the employer must use lockout, unless the employer can demonstrate that use of a tagout system will provide full employee protection. If an energy-isolating device is not capable of being locked out, the employer must use a tagout system.

For full employee protection, when a tagout device is used on an energy-isolating device, the device must be attached at the same location that the lockout device would have been attached, and the employer must demonstrate that the tagout device will provide a level of safety that is equivalent to that of a lockout system.

OSHA defines equipment that is "capable of being locked out" as that designed with a hasp or other fastener that a lock can go through or be affixed to, or that which has a locking mechanism built into it. A lock must be used if doing so will not require the employer to dismantle, rebuild, replace, or permanently alter the equipment's switch that turns the equipment on and off. For example, some valves and breakers are not designed to be locked, but they can be secured with chains, blocking braces, or wedges, all of which can be locked, according to OSHA.

In addition, the standard requires that when switches, circuit breakers, or other such devices are installed in a single cabinet or box, employers tag the specific switch or device, not the cabinet or box. All major replacement, repair, renovation, or modification of machines or equipment and all new machine or equipment installations must be designed to accept lockout devices.

Locks/tags

Locks, tags, chains, wedges, key blocks, adapter pins, self-locking fasteners, or other devices must be provided by the employer for isolating, securing, or blocking of machines or equipment from energy sources. Lockout/tagout devices must be singularly identified, must be the only devices used for energy control, and must not be used for other purposes.

Lockout/tagout devices also must

- be durable and capable of withstanding exposure to the environment. Tagout devices must be able to withstand weather conditions.

- be standardized within the facility in color, shape, or size. For tagout devices, print and format must be standardized as well.

- be substantial enough to prevent removal without the use of excessive force or unusual techniques—this especially applies to lockout devices. Tagout devices and the means to attach them must be substantial enough to prevent inadvertent or accidental removal.

- identify the employee applying the devices.

Tagout devices must warn against hazardous conditions if the machine or equipment is energized and must include appropriate warnings such as "Do Not Start," "Do Not Open," "Do Not Close," "Do Not Energize," and "Do Not Operate."

Training

Employees must be trained to understand the energy-control program and have the knowledge and skills needed for safe application, usage, and removal of energy controls. The employer must have written certification that each employee has received training. When tagout systems are used, employees must be trained to know that tags

- do not provide physical restraint and are essentially warning devices

- may provide a false sense of security

- must not be removed without authorization, and must never be bypassed, ignored, or otherwise defeated

- must be legible and understandable by all employees in the area

- must be made of materials that will withstand the environmental conditions around it

- must be securely attached to energy-isolating devices so that they cannot be inadvertently or accidentally removed

Retraining

Employers are required to provide retraining to maintain employee proficiency and when introducing any new or revised control methods and procedures. Retraining of authorized and affected employees also must be provided when

- there is a change in job assignments
- a new hazard is introduced due to a change in machines, equipment, or process
- there is a change in the energy-control procedures
- a periodic inspection by the employer reveals inadequacies in the company procedures or in the knowledge of the employees

Application of controls

The application of energy-control devices and the implementation of a lockout/tagout system must meet certain criteria under the OSHA standard (29 CFR 1910.147[d]). These requirements include the following:

- Only authorized employees may create the lockout/tagout systems
- Affected employees must be notified by the employer or authorized employee before the application and after the removal of the controls from the machine or equipment
- The authorized or affected employee who turns off a machine or equipment must be knowledgeable about the type and magnitude of the energy to be controlled, its hazards, and the methods to control that energy
- The machine or equipment must be turned off or shut down using the procedures required by the standard

- All energy-isolating devices needed to control the energy to the machine or equipment must be located and operated to isolate the machine or equipment from the energy sources

- Lockout/tagout devices must be affixed to each energy-isolating device by the authorized employee

- Lockout devices must be affixed so that the energy-isolating devices will remain in a "safe" or "off" position

- Tagout devices also must be affixed so that they clearly indicate that operation or movement of energy-isolating devices is prohibited

After the application of the controls, all potentially hazardous stored or residual energy must be relieved, disconnected, restrained, or rendered safe.

Before starting maintenance and/or servicing activities, the authorized employee must verify that isolation and de-energization of the machine or equipment is complete.

Release of lockout/tagout

Before lockout or tagout devices are removed and energy is restored to the machine or equipment, the authorized employee must ensure that it is safe to do so (29 CFR 1910.147[e]). To accomplish that, the OSHA standard requires the following:

- The work area must be inspected to ensure that nonessential items have been removed and the machine or equipment is operationally intact.

- All employees must be cleared from the area and safely positioned. All affected employees also must be notified that the lockout/tagout devices have been removed.

- Each lockout/tagout device must be removed from each energy-isolating device by the authorized employee who applied the devices.

Other requirements

Temporary removal of lockout/tagout

In situations where lockout/tagout devices must be removed temporarily to test or position the machine or equipment, specific actions must be taken (29 CFR 1910.147[f]). The following actions, in sequence, are required:

- Clear the machine of tools, materials, and other nonessential items
- Clear employees from the area
- Remove the lockout/tagout device
- Energize and proceed with testing and positioning
- De-energize all systems and reapply energy-control measures (lockout/tagout) to continue the servicing and/or maintenance work

Use of outside personnel

When outside personnel are engaged in servicing and/or maintenance work, the on-site employer and the outside employer must inform each other of their respective lockout/tagout procedures.

The on-site employer's personnel must understand and comply with the restrictions and prohibitions of the outside employer's energy-control procedures.

Service and maintenance

When service and/or maintenance is performed by a crew, craft, or other group, they must use procedures that afford employee protection that is equivalent to that of an individual lockout/tagout system.

Ensuring continuity of protection

Specific procedures must be used during shift or personnel changes to ensure the continuity of lockout/tagout protection.

Enforcement

An employer's method of enforcing the energy-control program, as well as compliance with specific requirements of the standard, will be evaluated by OSHA compliance officers. The compliance officer may ask the employer for any hazard analysis or any other basis on which the program related to the standard was developed. Although this is not a requirement, it aids in determining the adequacy of the program. Compliance officers also will ask for

- certification of periodic inspections
- certification of training
- written procedures that detail the methods used for control of hazardous energy, including shutdown, equipment isolation, lockout/tagout application, release of stored energy, and verification of isolation

The written procedure must identify the specific types of energy to be controlled. In instances where a common procedure is to be used, the specific equipment covered by the common procedure must be identified at least by type and location. The identification of the energy to be controlled may be by magnitude and type of energy.

When evaluating employee-training programs, an OSHA compliance officer will interview a sampling of employees to verify that they have been properly instructed in the purpose and use of the energy-control procedures.

If deficiencies are identified, the compliance officer will evaluate the employer's compliance with specific requirements of the standard and

- evaluate compliance with the requirements for periodic inspection of procedures.
- ensure that the person who performs the periodic inspection is an authorized employee who does not use the procedure being inspected.

- evaluate compliance with retraining requirements that result from the periodic inspection of procedures and practices, or from changes in equipment/processes.

- evaluate the employer's procedures for assessment and correction of deviations or inadequacies identified during periodic inspections of the energy-control procedure.

- identify the procedures for release from lockout/tagout, including replacement of safeguards, machine or equipment inspection, and removal of nonessential tools and equipment; safe positioning of employees; removal of lockout/tagout devices; and notification of affected employees that servicing and maintenance are completed.

- ensure that when a group lockout or tagout is used, it affords a level of protection equivalent to individual lockout or tagout. The company must ensure that no employee affixes a personal lockout/tagout device for another employee. Group lockout/tagout procedures must be tailored to the specific operation and may be unique in the manner that employee protection from the release of hazardous energy is achieved.

Some other more specific provisions that an employer should be aware of include the following:

- The standard also applies to high-intensity electromagnetic fields. Electromagnetic devices must be de-energized and held off whenever workers are present within a high-intensity ambient field.

- Servicing/maintenance of fire alarm and extinguishing systems and their components do not have to meet the standard if the workers performing the maintenance are protected from the unexpected release of hazardous energy by appropriate alternative measures.

- Minor tool changes and adjustments and other minor servicing activities that take place during normal operations are not covered by this standard if

    - they are routine, repetitive, and integral to the use of equipment for production.

    - work is performed using effective alternative protective measures.

- the exclusion of plug- and cord-connected electric equipment from the standard applies only when the equipment is unplugged and the plug is under the exclusive control of the employee performing the service and/or maintenance. The plug must be physically in the possession of the employee, in arm's reach and line of sight of the employee, or have a lockout/tagout device affixed on the plug.

- When lockout is used, the employer's periodic inspection will include a review of the responsibilities with the authorized employee who carries out the procedure. Group meetings between the authorized employee who is performing the inspection and all authorized employees who carry out the procedure are considered by OSHA to constitute compliance. When tagout is used, the employer must conduct this review with each affected and authorized employee.

- Energy-control procedures used less frequently than once a year need only be inspected when used.

Machine guarding (1910.212)

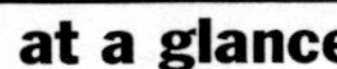

at a glance

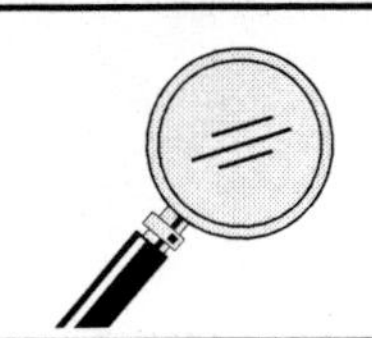

Guarding must be provided to protect employees from hazards at point of operation, flying chips, and sparks.

Machine guarding must be provided to protect employees in the machine area from hazards such as those created by point-of-operation, ingoing nip points, rotation parts, flying chips, and sparks. The guard must be such that it does not offer an accident hazard itself (29 CFR 1910.212[a][1] and [2]).

The point-of-operation guarding device must be so designed as to prevent the operator from having any part of the body in the danger zone during the operating cycle (29 CFR 1910.212[a][3][ii]).

Special supplemental hand tools for placing and removing material must permit handling of material without the operator placing a hand in the danger zone (29 CFR 1910.212[a][3][iii]).

Some of the machines that usually require point-of-operation guarding are guillotine cutters, shears, alligator shears, power presses, milling machines, power saws, jointers, portable power tools, and forming rolls and calendars (29 CFR 1910.212[a][3][iv]).

Fixed machinery

Machines designed for a fixed location must be securely anchored to prevent walking or moving or designed in such a manner that they will not move in normal operation (29 CFR 1910.212[b]).

Medical first aid (1910.151)

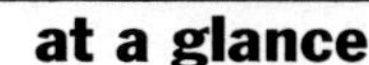

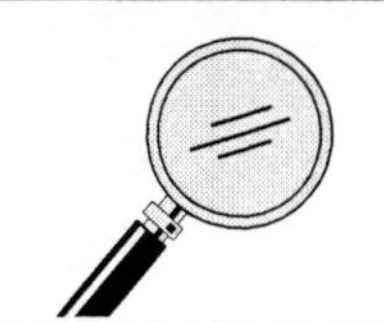

Employers must ensure the ready availability of medical personnel for advice and consultation on matters of occupational health. First-aid supplies shall be maintained for use by trained personnel.

The employer must ensure the ready availability of medical personnel for advice and consultation on matters of occupational health (29 CFR 1910.151[a]). When a medical facility for treatment of injured employees is not available in near proximity of the workplace, a person or persons must be trained to render first aid. First-aid supplies shall be maintained for use by trained personnel (29 CFR 1910.151[b]).

Mercury

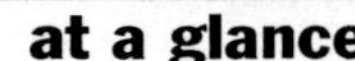

at a glance

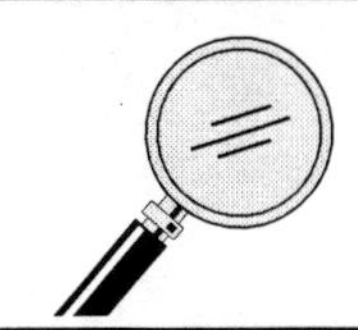

Mercury is regulated under OSHA's air-contaminants standard 1910.1000 through PELs. The EPA has additional controls.

Elemental mercury is a highly toxic, silvery, odorless, heavy liquid that vaporizes easily at room temperature. Inhalation is the major route of occupational exposure to mercury, but it also may be absorbed through the skin.

Mercury may be found in many forms in laboratory facilities. It may be used as a component in equipment, such as thermometers. Mercury is also an ingredient in chemicals. Mercury salts, for example, are contained in certain pathology fixatives and stains.

Organic mercury can be divided into two chemical groups: aryl compounds and alkyl compounds. Aryl compounds are sometimes contained in disinfectants used in laboratories. Alkyl compounds, such as methylmercury, are used in agricultural pesticides and fungicides. Organic mercury also has been used in the manufacture of some latex paints.

Adverse health effects

Inhalation of high concentrations of mercury vapor for relatively brief periods can cause acute health effects such as severe respiratory irritation, pneumonitis, bronchitis, chest pain, difficulty breathing, fever, coughing, stomatitis, gingivitis, salivation, and diarrhea.

Chronic effects from long-term exposure to low levels of mercury may include tremors, neuropsychiatric disturbances, and loss of appetite. Mercury also has been reported as a cause of sensitization dermatitis.

OSHA requirements and exposure limits

Employers are required under OSHA's air-contaminants standard to keep employee exposure to mercury within certain limits. The currently listed PEL for mercury is a ceiling of 0.1 mg/m^3.

A new set of exposure limits for mercury was issued by OSHA as part of the 1989 revisions to the air-contaminants standard. That regulatory attempt was nullified by a federal court. Had it not been defeated, however, it would have established PELs that included an eight-hour TWA of 0.05 mg/m^3 for mercury vapor, a ceiling limit of 0.1 mg/m^3 for inorganic mercury and aryl compounds, and an eight-hour TWA of 0.01 ppm and a STEL of 0.03 mg/m^3 for organic mercury. The 1989 revisions also required employers to take specific steps to protect employees from skin absorption. Many safety experts recommend that employers continue to comply with those exposure limits wherever possible.

Exposure limits for mercury also have been developed by NIOSH and the ACGIH. NIOSH recommends an exposure limit for inorganic mercury of 0.05 mg/m^3 as a 10-hour TWA. ACGIH recommends a TLV TWA for mercury alkyl compounds of 0.01 mg/m^3 and a STEL of 0.03 mg/m^3. The TLV TWA for all forms except alkyl vapor is 0.05 and 0.1 mg/m^3 for aryl and inorganic compounds.

Employers are required under the air-contaminants standard to enable engineering or administrative controls to keep exposure to mercury within permissible limits. Only in cases where such controls are not feasible may PPE and other measures be relied upon to meet the PELs.

Environmental monitoring

Mercury vapors can be measured with a direct-reading colorimetric dosimeter, diffusion tubes, mercury vapor analyzer or "sniffer," or charcoal tubes impregnated with iodine. Particulate contamination can be collected on a filter for subsequent analysis.

General exposure controls

Because mercury can be absorbed via inhalation and through the skin, it is important to protect employees from both routes of exposure. Wherever possible, ventilation systems should be installed to prevent the accumulation or recirculation of mercury vapor into the workroom.

Skin contact with elemental mercury, mercury solutions, and vapor should be prevented through the use of engineering controls, work practices, and PPE such as gloves or coveralls.

Preventing spills

In laboratories facilities, the greatest risk of occupational exposure to mercury occurs when there is an accidental spill. Such exposures usually happen when thermometers are broken during routine handling, sterilization, or centrifugation. Mercury spills also can present a risk to visitors and other individuals in the spill area.

Substitution of nonmercury medical devices, such as electric thermometers, is a simple and effective way to eliminate this risk. Another means of reducing the risk is to use devices that are less likely to be broken.

Spill cleanup procedures

Mercury has unique physical properties that make it difficult to control in the event of a spill. If not contained, spilled mercury can accumulate in the carpeting, on floors, and on other surfaces such as porous laboratory sinks and counters. Unnoticed accumulations have been discovered under rugs and floorboards and in the clothing of workers in laboratories. Employers may find it helpful to remove rugs and install seamless floors in areas where spills are more likely to occur.

All employees, especially those who handle mercury-containing equipment, should be trained in emergency procedures to follow in the event of a spill. The emergency plan should be posted and should cover cleanup procedures, PPE, and use of respirators. Mercury spill kits should be provided and kept handy for use in an emergency.

Other recommendations include the following:

- Clean up spills promptly using special mercury vacuum cleaners and a water-soluble mercury decontaminant.
- Wear disposable PPE, such as gowns, gloves, shoe covers, splash-proof goggles, and respirators, when cleaning up spills.
- Wash hands and skin thoroughly and do not eat, drink, or apply lip balm when handling mercury.
- Clearly post all spill areas and cordon them off until adequate cleanup has been accomplished. If the spill is extensive, remove patients and noncleanup personnel from the area.
- Use a mercury "sniffer" to more accurately determine whether cleanup is complete, rather than relying on a visual inspection.

Mercury wastes should be recycled or disposed of in accordance with EPA regulations (40 CFR 261.24).

Past contamination

Mercury's tendency to accumulate in hidden areas and remain undetected in the environment makes it a potential hazard even in places where it is no longer used or where current controls are adequate.

Some employers find it helpful to use a mercury "sniffer" to detect the substance in areas where it may not be visible to the eye. Laboratories where spills or improper use may have occurred in the past are likely sites of contamination.

Personal protective equipment (1910.132)

at a glance

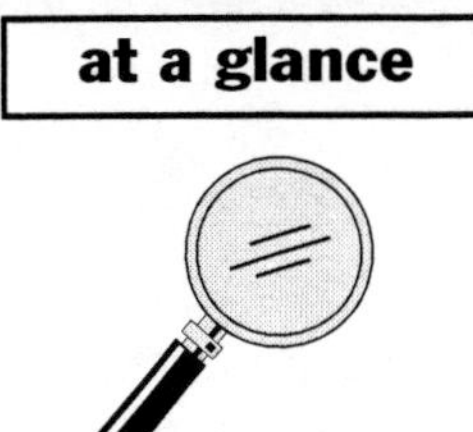

The PPE standard addresses general requirements for special equipment and coverage to protect workers from exposure to various elements, including disinfectants, radiation, medical waste, hazardous drugs, and asbestos. Specific requirements also fall under the respiratory-protection standard (1910.134).

Employers are required to provide and ensure that employees wear PPE wherever exposure to hazardous physical, chemical, or biological agents can cause injury or other impairments through inhalation, absorption, or physical contact, according to OSHA (29 CFR 1910.132). Required PPE must be maintained in a sanitary and reliable condition. Defective or damaged PPE may not be used.

Employers are required to conduct a hazard assessment to determine whether hazards that warrant use of PPE are present in the workplace. PPE includes protective equipment for the eyes, face, head, and extremities; protective clothing; respiratory devices; and protective shields and barriers. Respirators, if provided, should be properly fitted and provided as part of a written respiratory-protection program.

PPE may not be used as a substitute for feasible engineering, work-practice, or administrative controls (although its use may be relied upon during periods when engineering controls are being installed). Rather, it should be used in conjunction with these controls to provide for employee safety and health in the workplace.

Responsibility to provide and pay for PPE

OSHA generally requires employers to provide and pay for PPE necessary for the worker to perform the job safely and in compliance with OSHA standards.

Where equipment is personal in nature and is usable by workers off the job, however, the matter of who pays for the equipment may be left to labor-management negotiations.

Examples of PPE that is personal in nature and often used away from the work site include non-specialty safety glasses, safety shoes, and cold-weather outerwear.

Examples of PPE that would not normally be used away from the work site include respirators, specialty glasses and gloves, specialty foot protection, face shields, and rubber gloves.

Failure of the employer to pay for PPE that is not personal and not used away from the job is a violation and will be cited by OSHA.

In cases where employees provide their own PPE, the OSHA standard requires employers to ensure the adequacy, maintenance, and sanitation of the equipment.

Hazard-assessment requirements

Employers are required by OSHA to assess the workplace to determine whether hazards that necessitate the use of PPE are present or are likely to be present. If so, the employer is required to do the following:

- Select and have employees use the types of PPE that will protect employees from the hazards identified in the assessment
- Communicate selection decisions to each affected employee
- Select PPE that properly fits each affected employee

Certification

Verification that the workplace-hazard assessment has been performed must be maintained through a written certification that identifies the workplace evaluated, the person certifying that the evaluation has been performed, and the date(s) of the hazard assessment. The certification also must identify the document as a certification of hazard assessment.

Grandfathering of hazard assessments

According to an OSHA enforcement directive issued June 16, 1995, a hazard assessment conducted prior to July 5, 1994 (the initial effective date of the requirement) may be used to comply if the prior assessment meets all current requirements. An employer also may rely upon a hazard assessment conducted by a previous employer for the same work site, provided that it meets current requirements and that job conditions have not substantially changed. If an employer relies on a prior hazard assessment, the certification may contain the date on which the employer determined the prior assessment was adequate, rather than the date of the actual assessment.

Eye and face protection

Appropriate eye or face protection is required wherever there is a possibility of injury from flying particles, molten metal, liquid chemicals, acids or caustic liquids, chemical gases or vapors, or potentially injurious light radiation (29 CFR 1910.133).

Employees must use eye protection that provides side protection when there is a hazard from flying objects. Detachable side protectors (e.g., clip-on or slide-on side shields) are acceptable.

For protection from injurious light radiation, equipment must have filter lenses that have a shade number appropriate for the work being performed.

Employees who wear prescription lenses are required to wear eye protection that incorporates the prescription in the design, or eye protection that can be worn over the prescription lenses without disturbing their proper position (e.g., goggles).

OSHA also requires that eye and face protection meet performance standards developed by ANSI. The following specifics apply:

- If purchased after July 5, 1994, devices must comply with ANSI standard Z87.1-1989, "American National Standard Practice for Occupational and Educational Eye and Face Protection"

- If purchased before July 5, 1994, devices must comply with ANSI standard Z87.1-1968, "USA Standard for Occupational and Educational Eye and Face Protection"

Eye and face protection must be clearly marked to facilitate identification of the manufacturer.

Supervisors and visitors to the work area also must wear required protective gear.

Hand protection

Employers are required by OSHA to select and require employees to use appropriate hand protection when employees' hands are exposed to hazards such as those from skin absorption of harmful substances, severe cuts or lacerations, severe abrasions, punctures, chemical burns, thermal burns, and harmful temperature extremes (29 CFR 1910.138).

Employers are required to base the selection of the appropriate hand protection on an evaluation of its performance characteristics relative to the task to be performed, conditions present, duration of use, and the hazards and potential hazards identified.

Examples of situations where gloves and/or arm protectors may be required include tasks where workers handle objects with sharp edges or have potential contact with chemicals or infectious substances. Gloves and/or arm protectors also may be used to prevent burns or provide shielding from radiation produced by lasers and other devices.

The bloodborne-pathogens standard requires laboratory workers to wear gloves to prevent exposure to blood or OPIM. Workers who are allergic to commonly used latex gloves must be provided with an appropriate alternative.

Head protection

Protective head coverings, such as hard hats or helmets, are required in situations where workers may be injured by falling or flying objects (29 CFR 1910.135).

Protective helmets designed to reduce electrical-shock hazard must be worn by employees when near exposed electrical conductors that could contact the head. Head protection must comply with ANSI standards as detailed in the OSHA regulation.

Foot protection

Employees are required to wear protective footwear when working in areas where feet are exposed to electrical hazards and where there is a danger of foot injuries due to falling and rolling objects or a danger of objects piercing the sole (29 CFR 1910.136).

Safety shoes should be worn particularly where heavy materials or parts are handled and during shipping and receiving operations. Appropriate footwear with good traction should be worn for wet or slippery areas.

Aprons and leggings

Aprons and leggings may be necessary for some work activities, depending on the nature of the hazard.

Electrical protective equipment

Electrical protective equipment such as insulating blankets, matting, covers, line hose, gloves, and sleeves made of rubber must meet design, performance, and workmanship requirements detailed in the OSHA standard (29 CFR 1910.137).

Such equipment must be maintained in a safe and reliable condition. It should be stored away from light, temperature extremes, excessive humidity, ozone, and other injurious substances and conditions.

All insulating equipment must be inspected for damage before each day's use and following any incident that can reasonably be suspected of having caused damage. Damaged equipment may not be used. Repaired equipment must be tested in accordance with the standard's requirements before use by an employee.

Hearing protection

Employees must be provided with hearing-protection devices and directed to wear them wherever noise levels exceed limits allowed by OSHA.

Employee training

Employers must provide training to each employee who is required to use PPE (29 CFR 1910.132).

Employees must be trained to know the following:

- When PPE is needed
- What equipment is needed
- How to put on, take off, adjust, and wear the equipment
- The limitations of the equipment
- The proper care, maintenance, useful life, and disposal of the PPE

Employees must demonstrate an understanding of the specified training and the ability to use PPE properly before being allowed to perform work that requires its use.

In determining whether an employee has the required knowledge and skill, the employer may rely on training provided by a previous employer or the knowledge and ability, gained through prior experience, to use PPE properly.

Written certification

The OSHA standard requires the employer to provide written certification that each affected employee has been trained and understands the training. The certification should include the name of each employee trained, the date of the training, and the subject of the certification.

If the employer relies on training provided by another employer to an employee prior to July 5, 1994, or relies on the employee's prior experience, the certification may contain the date that the employer determined that the prior training was adequate, rather than the date of the actual training.

Retraining may be required if changes in the workplace or in the types of PPE render previous training obsolete. When an employer has reason to believe that any affected employee who already has been trained does not have the understanding and skill required, the employer must retrain the employee.

Respiratory protection

Laboratory workers often are exposed in the course of their work to airborne contaminants, physical hazards, and biological agents. OSHA requires employers to use engineering controls to prevent occupational diseases caused by breathing air contaminated with materials such as harmful dusts, fumes, mists, gases, sprays, and vapors. Where effective engineering controls are not feasible or while they are being installed, respirators should be used in accordance with requirements of OSHA's respiratory-protection standard (29 CFR 1910.134).

The standard requires employers to establish or maintain a respiratory-protection program to protect their respirator-wearing employees. The standard contains requirements for the following:

- Program administration
- Work site–specific procedures
- Respirator selection
- Employee training

- Fit testing
- Medical evaluation
- Respirator use
- Respirator cleaning, maintenance, and repair

The standard also simplifies respirator requirements for employers by deleting respiratory provisions in other OSHA health standards that duplicate those in the standard and by revising other respirator-related provisions to make them consistent. In addition, the standard addresses the use of respirators in IDLH atmospheres.

The standard includes detailed protocols for performing fit tests and lists the topics in which respirator users must be trained. It also contains provisions that address skin and eye irritation, both of which must be considered in respirator selection.

In the final rule for the revised respiratory-protection standard, OSHA redesignated the original text found at 29 CFR 1910.134 as 29 CFR 1910.139, "Respiratory protection for M. tuberculosis." For workers who are required to wear respirators for protection against tuberculosis, the requirements of 29 CFR 1910.139 apply.

To ensure uniform enforcement of the respiratory-protection standard, OSHA has issued guidelines to assist compliance officers while conducting inspections in workplaces where the standard may apply.

According to the compliance directive, whether an employer has created required engineering or work-practice controls, the employer may be issued a citation for failure to provide respirators when employees are exposed to hazardous levels of air contaminants. The employer must provide the correct type of respirator for the substance and level of exposure involved.

OSHA also added a chapter to its technical manual in 1999 to provide guidance on respiratory-protection issues for the agency's compliance inspectors.

Radiation (1910.1096 [ionizing] and 1910.97 [non-ionizing])

at a glance

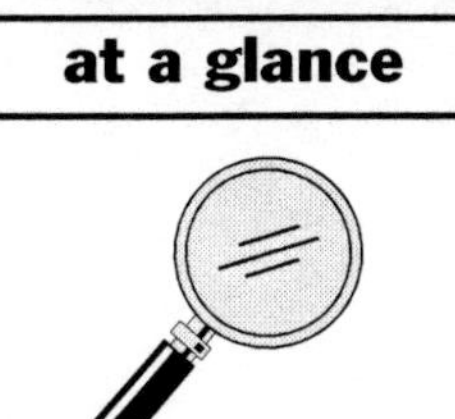

OSHA covers employee exposure to ionizing radiation sources not regulated by the NRC, such as x-ray equipment, accelerators, electron microscopes, and naturally occurring radioactive materials such as radium. Exposure to radio-frequency/microwave radiation is covered under the non-ionizing standard.

Employees in the healthcare environment may have exposure to both ionizing and non-ionizing sources of radiation. Ionizing radiation is produced artificially by atomic accelerators, such as x-ray machines, or naturally by the decay of radioactive material, such as may be found in radiopharmaceuticals or radioactive medical implants. Non-ionizing radiation is generated by sources such as ultraviolet lamps, lasers, ultrasound devices, and microwave ovens.

Ionizing radiation generally is thought to present the most severe potential health risk. Over-exposure can cause acute effects that range from radiodermatitis to shock, ulcerations, and death. Chronic effects may include an increased risk of cancer, cataracts, and sterility.

Responsibility for regulating worker exposure to ionizing radiation is shared by OSHA and the NRC. Generally, the NRC licenses and regulates the use of radioactive materials, while OSHA regulations cover hazards produced by x-ray machines and other types of atomic accelerators.

Exposure to non-ionizing radiation also should be monitored and controlled where possible. Potentially hazardous sources include ultrasound, ultraviolet and infrared light, and lasers. Adverse health effects may range from mild symptoms, such as headaches, to severe eye damage and skin burns.

Sources of radiation

Ionizing radiation is used for diagnostic radiology, including x-ray, fluoroscopy and angiography, dental radiography, and CAT scanners; therapeutic radiology; dermatology; nuclear medicine; and radiopharmaceutical laboratories.

Non-ionizing radiation may be generated by sources such as ultraviolet lamps, surgical lasers, ultrasound equipment, microwave ovens, and video-display terminals.

Regulation of hazards

OSHA generally has responsibility for ensuring the safety of workers who may be exposed to radiation and who are not protected by regulations issued by the NRC.

OSHA's jurisdiction includes employee exposures to radiation sources not regulated by the NRC, such as x-ray equipment, accelerators and accelerator-produced materials, electron microscopes and betatrons, and naturally occurring radioactive materials such as radium. Exposure to these sources is regulated under the standard for ionizing radiation (29 CFR1910.1096).

Exposure to radiofrequency/microwave radiation is regulated under the standard for non-ionizing radiation (29 CFR 1910.97). Other types of non-ionizing radiation (e.g., ultraviolet, ultrasound, and infrared) are not regulated under a specific OSHA standard. However, recommendations for exposure controls have been issued by other organizations, such as NIOSH and the ACGIH.

Many states have promulgated regulations to govern the use of sources of ionizing radiation. Check with your state OSHA department for more information.

Adverse health effects

Occupational exposure to radiation can produce both acute and chronic adverse health effects. The degree of damage depends upon which organs and tissues are radiated. Generally, the effects of radiation exposure are cumulative.

Ionizing radiation is a carcinogenic, teratogenic, and mutagenic agent. Localized occupational exposure can cause acute effects such as erythema or radiodermatitis. An acute radiation syndrome, where whole-body exposure exceeds 100 roentgens during a short period, occurs very rarely. Initial symptoms may include vomiting, diarrhea, and shock that progresses over a period of weeks to include fever and ulcerations. Death may result from severe bone marrow depression if the radiation exposure level is high. Chronic effects of exposure to ionizing radiation may include several types of cancers, lung and kidney fibrosis, cataracts, aplastic anemia, and sterility. Prenatal radiation exposure can cause various growth abnormalities and fetal death.

Non-ionizing radiation also may be hazardous. Some sources, such as visible radiation produced by lasers and ultraviolet radiation, can cause serious eye damage and skin burns. Radio frequency and microwave radiation have teratogenic effects and also may be carcinogenic. Overexposure to ultrasound radiation may produce symptoms such as tinnitus and, in some uses, physical damage to the hands of operators.

Ionizing radiation

The OSHA standard for ionizing radiation requires employers to monitor worker exposure to radiation and to keep such exposures within specified permissible limits.

Radiation covered under the standard includes x-rays, alpha rays, beta rays, gamma rays, neutrons, high-speed electrons, high-speed protons, and other atomic particles. The standard does not cover sound or radio waves, visible light, or infrared or ultraviolet light.

The standard provides the following definitions for determining hazard areas:

- **Restricted area**—any area to which access is controlled by the employer for the purpose of protecting individuals from exposure to radiation or radioactive materials

- **Radiation area**—any area accessible to personnel in which radiation exists at such levels that a major portion of the body could receive in any one hour a dose in excess of 5 millirem, or in any five consecutive days a dose in excess of 100 millirem

- **High-radiation area**—any area accessible to personnel in which radiation exists at such levels that a major portion of the body could receive in any one hour a dose in excess of 100 millirem

Exposure limits

Quarterly, employees in restricted areas may not receive a dose in excess of limits specified in the standard. Those dose or exposure limits are as follows:

- Whole body exposure (head and trunk, active blood-forming organs, lens of eyes or gonads)—1.25 rems
- Hands and forearms, feet and ankles—18.75 rems
- Skin of whole body—7.5 rems

An exception to these limits is available only in cases where (1) the dose to the individual's whole body does not exceed 3 rems during any calendar quarter and (2) the dose to the individual's whole body, when added to the accumulated occupational dose to the whole body, does not exceed 5(N-18) rems, where "N" equals the individual's age in years. In addition, the employer must maintain adequate past and current exposure records that show the addition of such a dose does not exceed authorized amounts.

Employers may not permit employees under 18 years of age to receive in any calendar quarter a dose in excess of 10% of the limits specified.

NRC regulations under 10 CFR 20 specify an occupational dose limit of 0.5 rem in a year for minors and for an embryo/fetus due to occupational exposure of a declared pregnant woman during the course of the pregnancy. The NRC has specified deep dose–equivalent monitoring criteria of 0.1 rem in a year for minors and for declared pregnant women.

Airborne radioactive material

Under the standard, employers may not allow employees to be exposed to airborne radioactive material in an average concentration in excess of the limits specified in Table 1 of Appendix B in NRC regulations at 10 CFR Part 20. Limits described in the table, which are based on a 40-hour work week, should be increased or decreased proportionately when the hours of exposure are greater than or less than 40. Employees under age 18 may be exposed to airborne concentrations no greater than those specified in Table II of Appendix B. Exposure is defined as occurring when an individual is present in an airborne concentration. In determining exposure, no allowance is made for particle size or the use of PPE.

Exposure monitoring

OSHA requires employers to evaluate the radiation hazards in their facility as necessary to ensure compliance with the standard. Such evaluation should include, where appropriate, a physical survey of the location of materials and equipment, and measurements of levels of radiation or concentrations of radioactive material present.

Personal monitoring equipment, such as dosimeters, generally must be worn in a restricted area by personnel who are likely to receive in any calendar quarter a radiation dose in excess of 25% of the applicable dose specified in the standard. This also applies to workers under age 18 who are likely to have exposure in excess of 5% of the value specified in the standard. Employee exposure levels must be analyzed and the results recorded.

Caution signs and labels

OSHA requires employers covered by the standard to post certain caution signs in hazard areas. The signs should portray the three-bladed radiation hazard symbol in magenta or purple on a yellow background.

Every radiation area must be conspicuously posted with a sign bearing the radiation caution symbol and the words "CAUTION: RADIATION AREA."

Every high-radiation area must be posted with a sign bearing the radiation symbol and the words "CAUTION: HIGH-RADIATION AREA." Each high-radiation area also must be equipped with a control device that either reduces the level of radiation below 100 millirems per hour upon entry or that sounds an audible alarm to notify the individual and the employer or supervisor of the entry. A high-radiation area established for 30 days or less need not have such a device.

Every airborne radioactivity area (as defined by Table 1 of Appendix B to 10 CFR Part 20) must be posted with a sign bearing the radiation symbol and the words "CAUTION: AIRBORNE RADIOACTIVITY AREA."

For storage of radioactive materials, signs bearing the radiation caution sign and the words "CAUTION: RADIOACTIVE MATERIALS" also should be posted at the following locations:

- Rooms or areas where natural uranium or thorium are used or stored in amounts that exceed 100 times the quantity specified in 10 CFR Part 20

- Rooms where radioactive materials other than natural uranium or thorium are stored in amounts in excess of 10 times the quantity specified in Appendix C to 10 CFR Part 20

Labels that bear the same information should be placed on each container in which natural uranium or thorium is transported, stored, or used in a quantity greater than 10 times that specified in Appendix C to 10 CFR Part 20. A label is not required where the concentration of material in the container does not exceed that specified in column 2 of Table 1 of Appendix B to 10 CFR Part 20 or for laboratory containers, such as beakers and flasks, when the user is present.

Sign-posting exceptions

An exception to the sign-posting requirement is allowed for rooms

- and other areas in on-site medical facilities where patients who contain radioactive materials are present, provided that there are personnel in attendance who take necessary precautions to prevent exposure of any individuals to radiation or radioactive material in excess of limits established by OSHA and the NRC

- that contain a sealed source of radiation, provided that the radiation level 12 inches from the surface of the source container or housing does not exceed 5 millirem per hour

- that contain radioactive materials for periods of less than eight hours, provided that the room is under the employer's control and that the materials are constantly attended by an individual who will take the precautions necessary to prevent exposure of any individual in excess of specified exposure limits

Evacuation warning signals

Immediate evacuation warning signals must meet a number of specifications under the standard. These include that the signal must be

- a specified frequency and not less than 75 decibels at every location where evacuation may be immediately necessary

- automatic, but designed so that false alarms do not occur so frequently that personnel may come to disregard the alarm

- connected to an automatically activated secondary power supply adequate to power all emergency equipment to which the signal is connected

Notification of incidents

Employers are required to report to OSHA within a specified period those radiation exposure incidents concerning employees not covered by NRC requirements.

Employers must immediately report any incident that may have caused or threatens to cause

- exposure of the whole body of any individual to 25 rems or more of radiation; exposure of the skin of the whole body of any individual to 150 rems or more of radiation; or exposure of the feet, ankles, hands, or forearms of any individual to 375 rems or more of radiation

- the release of radioactive material in concentrations that, if averaged over a period of 24 hours, would exceed 5,000 times the limit specified for such materials in Appendix B to 10 CFR Part 20

Within 24 hours, employers must report any radiation incident that may have caused or threatens to cause exposure of the whole body of any individual to 5 rems or more of radiation; exposure of the skin of the whole body of any individual to 30 rems or more of radiation; or exposure of the feet, ankles, hands, or forearms to 75 rems or more of radiation.

All such reports must be followed up with a written report that describes the extent of the personal exposure, levels of radiation and concentration of radioactive material involved, the cause of the exposure, and corrective steps taken or planned to prevent recurrence.

Employees must be provided written notice of the occurrence and extent of exposure incidents covered under these reporting requirements. The notice must contain the statement: "You should preserve this report for future reference."

Recordkeeping

Employers must maintain records of the radiation exposure of all employees for whom personnel monitoring is required under the standard. Employers must advise each of their employees about individual exposure at least annually. Employers are required to maintain these records indefinitely.

Disclosure

Employers must provide, upon request by a former employee, a written report of the employee's exposure to radiation as shown in records maintained under the standard. The report must be furnished within 30 days of the request and must cover each calendar quarter of the individual's employment involving exposure to radiation, unless a lesser period is requested by the employee. The report must contain the statement, "You should preserve this report for future reference."

Non-ionizing radiation

Non-ionizing radiation does not have enough energy to ionize atoms, but it vibrates and rotates molecules, causing heating. Non-ionizing radiation is classified by frequency and stated in units of hertz (Hz).

The only OSHA standard for non-ionizing radiation applies to electromagnetic radiation that originates from microwave ovens, radio stations, radar equipment, and certain other sources. The standard does not apply to the deliberate exposure of patients by, or under the direction of, healing practitioners.

UV radiation

Overexposure to UV radiation may result in skin burns and eye damage. Eye exposure is especially dangerous because the damage may not be apparent until six to eight hours after exposure. Long-term unprotected exposure may lead to partial vision loss, accelerated skin aging, and increased risk of skin cancer. OSHA does not have a standard regulating exposure to UV radiation. NIOSH has published recommendations. Threshold limit values for ultraviolet radiation also have been issued by ACGIH.

According to NIOSH, the best preventive approach to UV exposure is to provide a strong educational program and to issue protective glasses for potentially exposed workers. The use of shaded glass usually is sufficient to prevent damage to the eyes. Enclosures and shielding also may be used.

Visible radiation

Visible radiation sources include incandescent and fluorescent lighting and lasers.

Constant exposure to incandescent or fluorescent lighting may result in temporary effects such as visual fatigue and headaches. Glare can be reduced by properly positioning equipment, filters, or shields. Routine rest periods also are helpful.

Radiation from lasers can cause serious and irreversible eye damage and burns to the skin. OSHA generally requires personnel to wear PPE such as laser safety goggles to prevent exposures.

IR radiation

IR radiation is emitted by all objects with temperatures above absolute zero. The level of IR radiation increases with temperature.

Occupational exposure may occur during the use of heating and warming equipment in the kitchen and during procedures that involve lasers and thermography. Exposure hazards include acute skin burns and eye damage.

Eye protection with proper filters should be provided to workers for use in areas with IR radiation. Shielding and enclosures may be used to control exposure.

RF/microwave radiation

RF/microwave radiation may produce adverse effects, including potentially damaging alterations in cells. Thermal effects are in direct proportion to the field strength or power density. Effects associated with such radiation include neurological, behavioral, and immunological changes.

The OSHA standard for exposure to microwaves is 10 mW/cm^2. In addition, both ANSI and ACGIH have published guidelines for occupational exposure. The FDA's Bureau of Radiological Health sets limits on the amount of radiation leakage that is allowed from microwave ovens during normal use.

Microwave ovens should be checked for leakage regularly, at least every three months. Ovens should be kept clean, especially the door seals.

In addition, NIOSH recommends that any area where RF/microwave radiation exposure exceeds permissible limits should be considered potentially hazardous. The area should be clearly identified, and warning signs should be posted. Interlocks may be used to prevent unauthorized entry. Basic protective measures include the use of shields and absorbing enclosures for equipment. PPE, such as gonad shields, protective suits, and wire-netting helmets, also may be used.

Ultrasound

According to NIOSH, exposure to ultrasound does not appear to pose a human health risk. However, exposure to audible high-frequency radiation above 10 kHz can result in nausea, headaches, tinnitus, pain, dizziness, and fatigue. Exposure to powerful sources of ultrasound may cause damage to peripheral nervous and vascular structures at the point of contact, particularly in the hand.

Currently no OSHA standard or NIOSH recommendation has been issued to limit workplace exposure to ultrasound. ACGIH, however, has adopted threshold limit values for permissible exposure to airborne upper sonic and ultrasonic acoustic radiation.

Exposure to ultrasonic vibration can be reduced by the use of enclosures and shields, according to NIOSH. Sound-isolating panels on ultrasonic equipment should be free of openings and should be isolated from the floor by rubber seals. Workers operating or repairing ultrasonic equipment should be provided with appropriate PPE selected on the basis of the task being performed and the likelihood of exposure to radiation above 10 kHz or contact with low-frequency sources.

Video display terminals (VDTs)

VDTs are a frequent source of worker complaints about eyestrain and back, neck, and arm discomfort related to physical stress.

These problems may be prevented or controlled with ergonomic measures such as proper adjustment of screens and keyboards, appropriate chair height, good lighting and use of glare screens, and frequent rest and stretch periods.

According to NIOSH, health data and radiation measurements indicate that VDTs do not appear to present a radiation hazard to operators or to developing fetuses of pregnant operators. However, reports of miscarriages and birth defects among VDT operators have persisted in recent years, and study of the issue has continued.

Recordkeeping (1904)

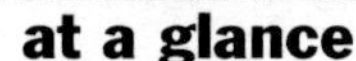

at a glance

The recordkeeping standard requires employers to maintain records of employees' occupational injuries and illnesses so OSHA can identify high-risk areas. It also requires employers to keep a log of all sharps injuries.

Laboratory employers may be required to maintain records of employees' occupational injuries and illnesses and make this data available to OSHA inspectors upon request (29 CFR 1904). The records provide employers with a means of evaluating the success of their safety and health activities and identifying high-risk areas to which attention should be directed.

OSHA requires employers with 11 or more employees to maintain injury and illness records at each of their establishments. Employers are required to record information about every occupational death, injury, or illness that results in days away from work, restricted work, job transfer, medical treatment beyond first aid, or loss of consciousness. A separate set of records must be kept for each establishment of any employer. Present and former employees and representatives of employees must be allowed access to records. Additional requirements apply to the maintenance and retention of records for medical surveillance, exposure monitoring, inspections, and other activities and incidents relevant to occupational safety and health (29 CFR 1910.1020).

Employers are required to report directly to OSHA any employee death or inpatient hospitalization of three or more employees that results from a work-related incident. Such reports must be made within eight hours by telephone, in person to the OSHA area office nearest to the incident, or by using the OSHA toll-free telephone number (800/321-6742). In states with approved safety and health plans, separate federal recordkeeping is not required because state requirements must be "substantially identical" to federal requirements.

On January 18, 2001, OSHA issued its revised recordkeeping rule that requires healthcare officials to record needlestick and sharps injuries on their work-related injury and illness logs. The revision is consistent with legislation that required OSHA to revise its bloodborne-pathogens standard to address such injuries. The rule, the majority of which took effect January 1, 2002, also addresses privacy concerns and simplifies some of OSHA's recordkeeping requirements. OSHA issued its compliance directive, CPL 2-0.131, on January 1, 2002.

OSHA reissued the final recordkeeping rule with amendments related to hearing loss and musculoskeletal disorders on July 1, 2002. On December 17, 2002, OSHA delayed until January 1, 2004 the requirements for recording hearing loss and musculoskeletal disorders on the OSHA 300 Log. On June 30, 2003, OSHA announced that it would not require employers to check a special box on the 300 Log for musculoskeletal injuries.

OSHA requires employers to prepare and maintain records of occupational injuries and illnesses to assist compliance, safety, and health officers in inspections and investigations. The recordkeeping system provides the basis for a statistical program that produces reliable injury and illness incidence rates and other measures. The information also helps employers identify many of the factors that cause injuries and illnesses in the workplace.

OSHA requires the following records to be maintained:

- All employers, regardless of the applicability of other recordkeeping requirements, must post the notice (poster) supplied by OSHA that informs employees of their rights under the law.

- Employers are required to keep an OSHA Form 300—the Log of Work-Related Injuries and Illnesses—and post an annual summary—OSHA 300-A—where employees generally read notices in the workplace from February 1 to April 30 every year. The summary should be completed after the Form 300 has been reviewed and verified for completeness and accuracy, and any deficiencies corrected. The summary must be certified by a company executive.

- OSHA Form 301 (the Injury and Illness Incident Report), which is the supplementary record of each injury and illness recorded in Form 300, must be maintained. In lieu of this OSHA form, a state workers' compensation form with equivalent information, or a similar form created by the employer with equivalent information, also may be kept.

Computer forms

Records may be kept on a computer system if your computer can produce equivalent forms when they are needed.

HIPAA and privacy concerns

OSHA has determined, in an August 2, 2004 letter of interpretation, that recordkeeping requirements for OSHA Form 300 do not violate the privacy requirements contained in the Health Insurance Portability and Accountability Act of 1996 (HIPAA). Except for privacy concern cases, as identified below, OSHA does not require employers to remove employees' names from Form 300 before providing access.

The employer may not enter an employee's name on the OSHA 300 Log when recording a privacy case. The employer must keep a separate, confidential list of the case numbers and employee names and must provide it to the government upon request. OSHA has identified privacy cases to include only the following situations:

- An injury or illness to an intimate body part or the reproductive system
- An injury or illness resulting from a sexual assault
- Mental illnesses
- HIV infection, hepatitis, or TB
- Needlestick injuries and cuts from sharp objects that are contaminated with another person's blood or OPIM
- Other illnesses, if the employee independently and voluntarily requests that his or her name not be entered on the log

Small employer exemption

Recordkeeping is not required for most small employers that employed no more than 10 full-time or part-time employees at any one time during the previous year. Some state safety and health laws may require regularly exempt small employers to keep injury and illness records. However, small employers are not exempt from the requirement to report any accident that results in one or more fatalities or the hospitalization of three or more employees.

Partially exempt industries

As of January 1, 2002, OSHA exempted "specific low hazard" industries, categorized by Standard Industrial Classification (SIC) codes, from the requirement to keep injury and illness records. Healthcare SIC codes exempt from recordkeeping include the following:

- SIC code 801: Offices and clinics of medical doctors—including ambulatory surgical centers, free-standing emergency medical centers, OB/GYN offices, and plastic surgeons

- SIC code 802: Offices and clinics of dentists—including dental surgeons, oral pathologists, endodontists, and orthodontists

- SIC code 803: Offices of osteopathic physicians

- SIC code 804: Offices of other health practitioners—including chiropractors, podiatrists, and occupational and physical therapists

- SIC code 807: Medical and dental laboratories—including x-ray, urinalysis labs, blood analysis labs, and analytic or diagnostic labs

- SIC code 809: Health and allied services—including kidney dialysis centers, birth control clinics (family planning), rehabilitation centers, blood banks, and respiratory therapy clinics

A complete list of partially exempt industries is available on the OSHA recordkeeping Web page at *www.osha.gov/recordkeeping/index.html.*

State occupational health and safety plans may not exempt industries from recordkeeping requirements. If your facility operates in a state with its own occupational safety and health plan, see Appendix A of this book for contact information.

All employers, including those partially exempted by industry classification, must report to OSHA any workplace incident that results in a fatality or the hospitalization of three or more employees.

Bureau of Labor Statistics (BLS) survey

OSHA requires employers to make periodic reports of deaths, injuries, and illnesses that have been recorded on the OSHA injury and illness records. This reporting is accomplished by the BLS, which selects several hundred thousand employers each year to participate in a national survey. The survey is conducted on the BLS Form 9300—Survey of Occupational Illnesses and Injuries. The OSHA injury and illness records maintained by employers in their establishments serve as the basis for the survey.

Employers that receive the survey are required to return the completed form within three weeks of receipt. Some small employers or employers in partially exempt industries may have to maintain records if they are selected to participate.

OSHA survey

OSHA conducts an annual survey of selected employers' injury and illness data, along with the number of workers employed and the hours they worked during designated periods. Establishment data collected by mail or other remote transmission are used to target agency resources to the more hazardous workplaces, as well as for rulemaking and periodic reassessment of regulations and standards.

The form used for the annual survey is OSHA Form 196-A or 196-B—Annual Survey Form. Form 196-A is sent to employers also selected for the BLS survey, and 196-B to those participating only in the OSHA survey. As with the BLS survey, injury and illness records maintained in the workplace serve as the basis for the OSHA survey, and employers have at least 30 days to respond to it.

Some small employers might be notified ahead of time by OSHA that they must maintain injury and illness records for participation in the annual survey.

OSHA Form 300

OSHA Form 300 is used to record injuries and illnesses for a calendar year. Every OSHA-recordable injury and illness must be recorded on an OSHA Form 300 (or equivalent) within seven calendar days from the time the employer learns of the injury or illness. Information requested on the form includes company name and establishment name and address. It also includes employee details such as name; occupation; department; description of injury or illness; extent of and outcome of injury; type, extent, and outcome of illness; and days away from work.

Days away from work include the number of calendar days that an employee is away from his or her job. Injury- and illness-related fatalities are to be included. Where there is a doubt as to whether an illness or injury is work-related, an entry should be made and can be canceled at a future time following a determination. This also applies to death, because it is often difficult to determine whether a fatal heart attack, for example, is work-related. If the fatal heart attack occurs at the workplace, it is to be recorded. Termination of employment or permanent transfers are to be identified with regard to illnesses.

The log of injuries and illnesses should be made available on request to any former or current employee or employee representative (e.g., a labor organization). Access to the log is limited to establishments where the employee is or has been employed.

The OSHA Form 300 must be retained for five years after the end of the year to which it relates. The forms must be available (normally at the establishment) for inspection and copying by representatives of OSHA, NIOSH, or state inspectors in states that have their own enforcement programs. If an establishment changes ownership, the new employer must preserve the records for the remainder of the five-year period. However, the new employer is not responsible for updating the records of the former owner.

If there are changes in the extent or outcome of an injury or illness, they must be recorded and a line struck through the previous entry.

OSHA Form 301

To supplement the log of work-related injuries and illnesses (OSHA Form 300), each establishment must maintain a record of each recordable work-related injury or illness. Workers' compensation, insurance, or other reports are acceptable as records if they include all facts listed or are supplemented to do so. If no suitable report is made for other purposes, OSHA Form 301 may be used, or the necessary facts can be listed on a separate sheet of plain paper.

Completed supplementary records must be present in the establishment within seven calendar days after the employer receives information that an injury or illness has occurred, and they must be available at reasonable times for examination by representatives of OSHA and the states with their own enforcement programs.

Supplementary records must contain at least the following:

- The employer's name, mailing address, and location, if different from mail address
- The employee's name, Social Security number, home address, age, gender, occupation, and department
- The location where the accident or exposure to occupational illness occurred, whether it was on the employer's premises, what the employee was doing when injured, and how the accident occurred

- A description of the injury or illness, including part of body affected, name of the object or substance that directly injured the employee, and date of injury or diagnosis of illness
- The name and address of the physician and, if the employee is hospitalized, name and address of the hospital
- The date of the report and the name and position of the person preparing it

Supplementary records must be retained for at least five years after the end of the year to which the records relate.

Exposures to bloodborne pathogens

Record all work-related exposures to blood or OPIM through events such as a needlestick, laceration, or splash. The person responsible for this recordkeeping must be knowledgeable about OSHA's recordkeeping requirements. For OSHA Form 300 recordkeeping purposes, an occupational bloodborne-pathogens-exposure incident is classified as an injury, because it is usually the result of an instantaneous event or exposure. To protect the employee's privacy, you may not enter the employee's name on the OSHA 300 Log. If the injured employee is later diagnosed with an infectious bloodborne disease, update the classification of the case on the 300 Log if the case results in death, days away from work, restricted work, or job transfer. The description also must be updated to identify the disease and the classification must be changed to an illness.

The revised bloodborne-pathogens standard also requires employers to keep a sharps-injury log. The log must contain a list of all needlestick injuries and the sharps devices involved in them.

If an employer meets the exemption for the OSHA recordkeeping rule, the employer does not have to maintain a sharps log. Dentists' offices and doctors' offices, for example, are not required to keep sharps logs, according to CPL 02-00-135—Recordkeeping Policies and Procedures Manual, December 2004.

Other recording criteria

The revised standard also includes specific recording criteria for the following:

- **Medical removal.** Record the case on the 300 Log if an employee is medically removed under the medical-surveillance requirements of an OSHA standard. The case must be entered as involving either days away from work or restricted work activity. If the medical removal is the result of a chemical exposure, check the "poisoning" column.

- **Hearing loss.** Check the "hearing loss" column on the 300 Log if an employee's hearing test reveals that

  - the employee has experienced an STS in hearing in one or both ears (averaged at 2000, 3000, and 4000 Hz).

  - the employee's total hearing level is 25 dB or more above audiometric zero (also averaged at 2000, 3000, and 4000 Hz) in the same ear(s) as the STS, which is considered a "significant" hearing loss. Employers are allowed to adjust for hearing loss caused by aging, to retest hearing to make sure the loss is persistent, and to seek medical advice to determine whether the hearing loss is work-related. A revised final rule governing hearing loss was published in the ***Federal Register*** December 17, 2002 (67 ***FR*** 77165).

- **TB.** Check the "respiratory condition" column on the 300 Log if an employee has been occupationally exposed to anyone with a known case of active TB and that employee subsequently develops a TB infection, as evidenced by a positive skin test or diagnosis by a physician or other licensed healthcare professional.

- **MSD.** There are no special criteria for determining which MSDs to record, according to OSHA. An MSD case is recorded using the same process you would use for any other injury or illness. If an MSD is work-related, is a new case, and meets one or more of the general recording criteria, record it.

Reporting

Report the fatality of one or more employees or the inpatient hospitalization of three or more employees as the result of a work-related incident within eight hours by telephone, in person to the OSHA area office nearest to the site of the incident, or by using the OSHA toll-free telephone number (800/321-6742). This requirement applies to fatalities or hospitalizations that occur within 30 days of an incident.

If the employer does not learn of a reportable incident at the time it occurs, the report to OSHA must be made within eight hours of the time that the employer learns of the incident.

Each fatality/hospitalization report must contain the following information:

- Name of establishment
- Location of incident
- Time of incident
- Number of fatalities or hospitalized employees
- Names of any injured employees
- Contact person and phone number
- Brief description of the incident

Small employers are not exempt from this requirement. According to OSHA, an employee is considered hospitalized when he or she is admitted to the hospital on an inpatient basis. Emergency room and all other forms of outpatient care are excluded from the reporting requirement.

MSDSs

Employers are required under the federal hazard-communication standard to maintain an MSDS for each hazardous chemical that is used in the workplace. MSDSs must be available to employees, their representatives, and OSHA and NIOSH, upon request. Employers also may be required by state law to make MSDSs available.

Tests, inspections, and maintenance checks

For certain types of equipment, OSHA allows employers to certify that safety tests and inspections of equipment have been conducted rather than requiring them to maintain detailed inspection records. Types of equipment for which certification is permitted in lieu of inspection records include manlifts; portable fire extinguishers; crane hooks, hoist chains, brakes, and ropes; mechanical power-press safeguards, clutches, and brakes; forging machine guards and point-of-operation protection devices; welding, cutting, and brazing equipment; shackles and hooks; and portable air receivers.

Instead of the detailed records, employers must prepare a certification record of a test, inspection, or maintenance check at the time the required work is done. The record must include the date on which the test, inspection, or maintenance check was performed; the signature of the person who performed the work; and an identifying name or number for the equipment or machinery that was inspected or tested.

Medical and exposure records

In addition to OSHA Form 300 and OSHA Form 100, the standard for access to employee exposure and medical records (29 CFR 1910.1020) requires employers to preserve and maintain exposure and medical records.

Individual health records must be kept in the EHS department. OSHA defines an employee medical record as one concerning the health status of an employee that is made or maintained by a physician, registered nurse, or other healthcare professional or technician. Each employee health record must be maintained for the duration of employment plus 30 years, unless a specific occupational safety and health standard requires a different period of time. Laboratory reports and worksheets only need to be kept for one year.

Employers also are required to maintain accurate records of certain potentially toxic or harmful physical agents that must be monitored or measured. Employers must advise employees promptly of any excessive exposure and of the corrective action taken. In certain cases, physical examinations and testing are required.

OSHA requires that employee exposure records be maintained for the duration of employment plus 30 years, and that employees or their designated representatives have a right to review their individual employee medical records and records describing employee exposures.

When employees request their exposure records, the employer is required to furnish them within 15 days. Employee representatives also may examine and copy a worker's exposure records. If prescribed procedures are followed, OSHA has the right to see exposure records.

Confidentiality

Employee health records must be treated with the level of confidentiality necessary to protect employee privacy. However, the employer must make the records available to the employee, or authorized representative, on employee request. Employees, or their representatives, have the right to examine and copy the results of exposure monitoring. The employee exposure record contains information about employee exposure, such as the following:

- Environmental monitoring, specific sampling results, the collection methodology, a description of the analytical and mathematical methods used, and a summary of other background data relevant to interpretation of the results obtained

- Biological monitoring results that directly assess the absorption of a hazard

- MSDSs or a hazard inventory that describes chemicals and identifies where and when they are used

Exemptions

The following types of records are exempt from the retention rule:

- Health insurance–claims records maintained separately from the employer's medical program and its records
- First-aid records of one-time treatment and subsequent observation
- Medical records of employees who have worked for less than one year for the employer (these need not be retained beyond the term of employment if they are provided to the employee upon termination)
- Records concerning voluntary employee-assistance programs (e.g., for alcohol, drug abuse, or personal counseling) if maintained separately from the employer's medical program and its records

Additional requirements

The records-access standard also includes the following provisions:

- The storage of information in any form—document, microfilm, x-ray, or automated data processing—is permitted, except that chest x-rays must be kept in their original state
- Employer trade secrets should conform with OSHA's hazard-communication standard
- Employee representatives (such as union representatives) must show an occupational-health need for requested records when seeking access to employee exposure records without consent

Employers are required to ensure access to the following:

- Pertinent exposure records by the exposed employee
- Fellow employees exposed or potentially exposed to similar job hazards
- Designated employee representatives

OSHA

Similar provisions apply to employees' medical records. However, for privacy interests, employee representatives are allowed access to the records only with written consent of the concerned employee. The records-access rule requires that employees be informed upon employment and annually thereafter of their rights of access to the records and the correct procedures for exercising those rights.

Recordable injuries and illnesses

A decision tree can be used to determine whether to record work-related injuries and illnesses. The steps are as follows:

1. Did the employee experience an injury or illness?
2. Is the injury or illness work-related?
3. Is the injury or illness a new case? (If the answer is no, update the previously recorded log entry, if necessary.)
4. Does the injury or illness meet the general recording criteria (death, days away from work, restricted work or transfer to another job, medical treatment beyond first aid, loss of consciousness, diagnosis of a significant injury/illness by a physician or other licensed healthcare professional), or the application to specific cases?

If you answer yes to all of these questions, record the injury or illness.

Determine whether a case has occurred

Normally, recognizing injuries and illnesses is simple, but some situations trouble employers. For example, if an employee is sent to or goes to a hospital for observation, the event is not recordable, provided that no medical treatment was given or no illness was recognized. Further, if symptoms from a previous injury or illness recur, no new entry should be made for the recurrence. However, if a previous injury is significantly aggravated by a new incident, such as a slip or fall, the incident should be recorded as a new case. If an occupational illness recurs as the result of new exposures to sensitizing agents, it should be recorded as a new case. In any event, the recurrence of symptoms of previous illnesses may require adjustment of previous entries to reflect possible changes in the extent of outcome of the particular case.

Establish that the illness or injury was work-related

If an event or exposure in the work environment either caused or contributed to the resulting condition or significantly aggravated a preexisting injury or illness, it is considered work-related. The work environment is defined as the establishment and other locations where one or more employees are working or are present as a condition of their employment. Work environment also includes equipment or materials used during the course of work. You are not required to record injuries and illnesses if the following exceptions specifically apply:

- The employee was present in the work environment as a member of the general public.
- The injury or illness involves signs or symptoms that surface at work but result solely from a non-work-related event or exposure that occurs outside the work environment.
- The injury or illness results solely from voluntary participation in a wellness program or in a medical, fitness, or recreational activity such as blood donation, physical examination, flu shot, exercise class, racquetball, or baseball.
- The injury or illness is solely the result of eating, drinking, or preparing food or drink for personal consumption, whether bought on-site or brought in. If the employee is made ill by food contaminated by workplace contaminants or gets food poisoning from food supplied by the employer, the case would be considered work-related.

- The injury or illness is solely the result of an employee performing personal tasks at the establishment outside of the employee's assigned work hours.
- The injury or illness is solely the result of personal grooming, is solely the result of self-medication for a non-work-related condition, or is intentionally self-inflicted.
- The injury or illness is caused by a motor vehicle accident on a company parking lot or access road while commuting to or from work.
- The illness is the common cold or flu. Contagious diseases such as TB, brucellosis, hepatitis A, or plague are considered work-related if the employee is infected at work.
- The illness is a mental illness. Mental illness will not be considered work-related unless the employee voluntarily provides the employer with an opinion from a physician or other licensed healthcare professional with appropriate training and experience stating that the mental illness is work-related.

Employees who travel on company business are considered to be engaged in work-related activities all the time they spend in the interest of the company, including such activities as going to and from customer contacts and client-related entertainment. However, an injury or illness would not be recordable if it occurred during normal living activities such as eating or sleeping, or during the time the employee deviates from a reasonably direct route of travel for vacation or other personal reasons. The employee would again be in the course of employment when he or she returns to the normal route of travel. When traveling employees check into a hotel, they establish a home base. Thereafter, their activities in that context are evaluated in the same way as those of nontraveling employees.

Recordkeeping and classifying illness and injury

An injury or illness is considered a new case if the employee has not previously experienced a recorded injury or illness of the same type that affects the same part of the body. If the employee has recovered from the same injury or illness but an event or exposure in the workplace caused the signs or symptoms to reappear, the case is considered new. When an employee experiences the signs or symptoms of a chronic work-related illness, do not consider each recurrence of signs or symptoms as a new case when they recur or continue in the absence of a workplace exposure. However, when an employee experiences the signs or symptoms or an injury or illness as a result of an event or exposure in the workplace, the episode must be treated as a new case.

General recording criteria

Any injury or illness is recordable if it results in any of the following:

- Death
- Days away from work
- Restricted work or transfer to another job
- Medical treatment beyond first aid
- Loss of consciousness
- A significant injury or illness diagnosed by a physician or other licensed healthcare professional

When an injury or illness involves one or more days away from work, record the injury or illness on the 300 Log and enter the number of calendar days away from work. Enter an estimate if the employee is out for an extended time, and then update the count later. Begin counting days away on the day after the injury or illness occurred.

When an injury or illness involves restricted work or job transfer but does not involve death or days away from work, record the injury or illness on the 300 Log and enter the number of restricted or transferred days in the restricted workdays column. Restricted work occurs when you keep the employee from performing one or more routine functions of his or her job or from working the full workday, or if a physician or other licensed healthcare professional recommends that the employee not perform certain functions or work a full day.

If a work-related injury or illness results in medical treatment beyond first aid, record it on the 300 Log. If the injury or illness did not involve death, one or more days away from work, one or more days of restricted work, or one or more days of job transfer, enter a check mark in the box for cases where the employee received medical treatment but remained at work.

Medical treatment

Medical treatment refers to the management and care of a patient to combat disease or disorder. Medical treatment does not include the following:

- Visits to a physician or other licensed healthcare professional solely for observation or counseling
- The conduct of diagnostic procedures, such as x-rays and blood tests, including the administration of prescription medications used solely for diagnostic purposes (e.g., eye drops to dilate pupils)
- First aid, as defined next

First aid

First aid includes the following complete list of treatments:

- Using a nonprescription medication at nonprescription strength (use of a nonprescription medication at prescription strength is considered medical treatment)
- Administering tetanus immunizations (other immunizations, such as Hepatitis B vaccine or rabies vaccine, are considered medical treatment)
- Cleaning, flushing, or soaking wounds on the surface of the skin
- Using wound coverings (such as bandages, Band-Aids®, gauze pads, etc.) or using butterfly bandages or Steri-Strips® (note that other wound-closing devices such as sutures, staples, etc., are considered medical treatment)
- Using hot or cold therapy

- Using any nonrigid means of support, such as elastic bandages, wraps, nonrigid back belts, etc. (note that devices with rigid stays or other systems designed to immobilize parts of the body are considered medical treatment)
- Using temporary immobilization devices while transporting an accident victim (e.g., splints, slings, neck collars, back boards, etc.)
- Drilling of a fingernail or toenail to relieve pressure, or draining fluid from a blister
- Using eye patches
- Removing foreign bodies from the eye using only irrigation or a cotton swab
- Removing splinters or foreign material from areas other than the eye by irrigation, tweezers, cotton swabs, or other simple means
- Using finger guards
- Using massages (note that physical therapy or chiropractic treatment are considered medical treatment)
- Drinking fluids for relief of heat stress

OSHA Recordkeeping Handbook

OSHA maintains a Recordkeeping Handbook on the Web that updates regulations and interpretations for recording and reporting occupational injuries and illnesses. The handbook presents many "what if . . ." situations for determining work-relatedness and reporting requirements. It is available at *www.osha.gov/recordkeeping/handbook/index.html.*

Respiratory protection (1910.134)

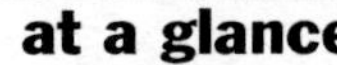
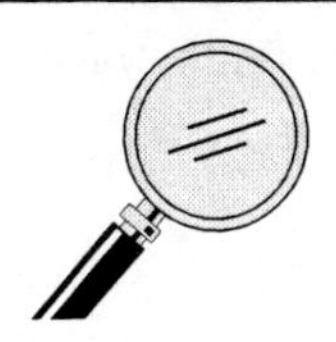

The respiratory-protection standard requires employers to provide respirators to protect employees from insufficient oxygen environments, harmful airborne substances, and diseases. Specific hazards related to TB are addressed in a compliance directive rather than in a separate standard. OSHA also refers to NIOSH respirator standards under 42 CFR 84 subpart K. .

In the course of their work, laboratory workers often are exposed to airborne contaminants, physical hazards, and biological agents. OSHA requires employers to use engineering controls to prevent occupational diseases caused by breathing air contaminated with such materials, including harmful dusts, fumes, mists, gases, sprays, and vapors. Where effective engineering controls are not feasible or while they are being installed, respirators should be used in accordance with the requirements of OSHA's respiratory-protection standard (29 CFR 1910.134).

The standard requires employers to establish or maintain a respiratory-protection program to protect their respirator-wearing employees. The standard contains requirements for the following:

- Program administration
- Work site–specific procedures
- Respirator selection
- Employee training
- Fit testing
- Medical evaluation
- Respirator use
- Respirator cleaning, maintenance, and repair

The standard also simplifies respirator requirements for employers by both deleting respiratory provisions in other OSHA health standards that duplicate those in the standard and revising other respirator-related provisions to make them consistent. In addition, the standard addresses the use of respirators in IDLH atmospheres, including interior structural firefighting.

The standard includes detailed protocols for performing fit tests and lists the topics in which respirator users must be trained. It also contains provisions that address skin and eye irritation, both of which must be considered in respirator selection.

In the final rule implementing its comprehensive respiratory protection standard, OSHA redesignated the original text found at 29 CFR 1910.134 as 29 CFR 1910.139, "Respiratory protection for M. tuberculosis." On December 31, 2003, OSHA withdrew the proposed TB standard, revoked 29 CFR 1910.139, and declared that all TB exposures fall under the 1998 revisions to 29 CFR 1910.134.

To ensure uniform enforcement of the respiratory-protection standard, OSHA has issued guidelines to assist compliance officers while conducting inspections in workplaces where the standard may apply.

According to the compliance directive, whether an employer has carried out required engineering or work-practice controls, the employer may be issued a citation for failure to provide respirators when employees are exposed to hazardous levels of air contaminants. The employer must provide the correct type of respirator for the substance and level of exposure involved.

OSHA also added a chapter to its technical manual in 1999 to provide guidance on respiratory-protection issues for the agency's compliance inspectors.

Respiratory-protection program

Under the standard, employers must develop a respiratory-protection program with work site–specific procedures and elements for required respirator use. The program must be administered by a suitably trained program administrator. In addition, certain program elements may be required for voluntary use to prevent potential hazards associated with the use of the respirator.

The program must be updated as necessary to reflect those changes in workplace conditions that affect respirator use. The employer must include in the program the following provisions:

- Procedures for selecting respirators for use in the workplace
- Medical evaluations of employees required to use respirators

- Fit-testing procedures for tight-fitting respirators
- Procedures for proper use of respirators in routine and reasonably foreseeable emergency situations
- Procedures and schedules for cleaning, disinfecting, storing, inspecting, repairing, discarding, and otherwise maintaining respirators
- To ensure adequate air quality, quantity, and flow of breathing air for atmosphere-supplying respirators
- Training of employees in the respiratory hazards to which they are potentially exposed during routine and emergency situations
- Training of employees in the proper use of respirators, including donning and removing, any limitations on their use, and their maintenance
- Procedures for regularly evaluating the effectiveness of the program

Program administrator

A respiratory-protection program administrator must be designated to oversee and evaluate the respirator program. The administrator must be suitably trained and have the appropriate accountability and responsibility to manage the full respiratory-protection program.

In its inspection procedures, OSHA clarifies that facilities with multiple work sites may have a program administrator at each work site, one program administrator for several sites, or one program administration for several similar sites, as long as the standard's requirements are met.

Respirator selection and use

Where respirators are required, respirators (and their associated requirements, such as fit testing and maintenance), training, and medical evaluations must be provided at no cost to the employee. If employers allow the voluntary use of respirators other than filtering facepieces, the costs of activities associated with ensuring that the respirator itself does not create a hazard, such as medical evaluations and maintenance, must be covered by the employer.

The employer must provide the correct type of respirator for the substance and level of exposure involved. If the employer provides the wrong kind of respirator, a citation may be issued for not providing an appropriate respirator, unless a substance-specific standard is applicable.

Respirators must be selected from a sufficient number of respirator models and sizes so that each respirator is acceptable to, and correctly fits, the user. Respirators must be certified by NIOSH and must be used in compliance with the conditions of certification.

Respirators fall into one of two general "fit" types:

- **Tight-fitting**—quarter masks, which cover the mouth and nose; half masks, which fit over the nose and under the chin; and full facepieces, which cover the face from the hairline to below the chin

- **Loose-fitting**—hoods, helmets, blouses, or full suits that cover the head completely

There also are two major classes of respirators:

- Air-purifying respirators, which remove contaminants from the air

- Atmosphere-supplying respirators, which provide clean breathing air from an uncontaminated source

In general, atmosphere-supplying respirators are used for more hazardous exposures.

The employer is required to develop standard procedures for respirator use. The procedures should include all information and guidance necessary for their proper selection, use, and care. Possible emergency and routine uses of respirators should be anticipated and planned for, according to the standard.

Employees are required to use the respirators in accordance with training and instructions received from the employer.

Where respirator use is not required,

- an employer may provide respirators at the request of employees or permit employees to use their own respirators, if the employer determines that such respirator use will not in itself create a hazard. If the employer determines that any voluntary respirator use is permissible, the employer must provide the respirator users with the information contained in Appendix D of 29 CFR 1910.134 ("Information for Employees Using Respirators When Not Required Under the Standard").

- the employer must establish those elements of a written respiratory-protection program necessary to ensure that any employee using a respirator voluntarily is medically able to use that respirator. The respirator must be cleaned, stored, and maintained so that its use does not present a health hazard to the user.

Respiratory hazards

Employers must identify and evaluate respiratory hazards in the workplace. The evaluation must include a reasonable estimate of employee exposures to respiratory hazards and an identification of any contaminant's chemical state and physical form.

Oxygen-deficient atmospheres and atmospheres that are not or cannot be estimated must be treated as IDLH environments. For other contaminants, conducting personal air monitoring is not explicitly required by the respirator standard, although it is the most reliable and accurate method of determining exposure. Under the standard, employers must determine whether the quantity, circumstances, and use of hazardous chemicals require further evaluation for respiratory hazards. MSDSs contain information about physical and chemical characteristics of hazards, primary routes of entry, and generally applicable control measures. OSHA adds that some MSDSs also include recommendations for appropriate respiratory protection. For chemicals that do present a potential respiratory hazard, employers can contact the chemical manufacturer for additional information about predicted exposure levels and methods to further control worker exposure.

Employers also are required to provide appropriate respirators as a result of changes in the workplace, such as change in equipment, process, products, or control measures that could result in new exposures.

Several workplace situations involve toxic substances and substances for which engineering controls may be inadequate to control exposures. Respirators are used in these situations as a backup method of protection. Substances that have been associated with death or serious incidents include carbon monoxide, trichloroethylene, carbon dioxide, chromic acid, coal tar, toxic metal fumes and dusts, sulfur dioxide, wood dust, and welding fumes. These substances cause adverse health effects that range from transient, reversible effects (such as irritation or narcosis) to disabling diseases such as silicosis and asbestosis, to death caused either by acute exposure or by a cancer resulting from chronic exposures. Respirators are available to protect against inhalation of these toxic substances.

Radiation

Airborne contaminants may be radioactive. Exposure to ionizing radiation can cause acute effects such as nausea and vomiting, malaise and fatigue, increased temperature, and blood changes. More severe delayed effects include leukemia, bone and lung cancer, sterility, chromosomal and teratogenic damage, shortened life span, cataracts, and radiodermatitis (i.e., a dry, hairless, red, atrophic skin condition that can include skin cracking and depigmentation). Respirators that protect against the inhalation of radioactive particles are commonly used by workers exposed to these hazards.

Bioaerosols

Respirators that protect against the inhalation of biological agents are widely used in laboratory and other workplace settings where exposure to such agents presents a hazard. Airborne contaminants that are alive or were released from a living organism may cause pulmonary effects, including rhinitis, asthma, allergies, hypersensitivity diseases, humidifier fever, and epidemics of infections such as colds, viruses, TB, and Legionnaires' Disease. Cardiovascular effects that manifest as chest pain and nervous system effects that manifest as headache, blurred vision, and impaired judgment have occurred in susceptible workers following exposure to bioaerosols.

Oxygen deficiency

Respirators also can provide protection from oxygen-deficient atmospheres. Human beings begin to suffer adverse health effects when the oxygen level of their breathing air drops below the normal atmospheric level. Below 19.5% oxygen by volume, air is considered oxygen-deficient. At concentrations of 16%–19.5%, workers engaged in any form of exertion rapidly can become symptomatic as their tissues fail to obtain the oxygen necessary to function properly. Increased breathing rates, accelerated heartbeat, and impaired thinking or coordination occur more quickly in an oxygen-deficient environment.

Several workplace conditions lead to oxygen deficiency. Simple asphyxiants, or gases that are physiologically inert, can cause asphyxiation when present in high enough concentrations to lower the oxygen content in the air. Other toxic or chemical asphyxiants can poison hemoglobin, cytochromes, or other enzyme systems. A number of asphyxiants are gases that can evolve from explosions, combustion, chemical reactions, or heating. A high-temperature electrical fire or arc-welding accident causing a complete flashover in an enclosed area can temporarily eliminate oxygen from that area.

Physiological burdens

In some cases, respirator use itself can cause illness and injury to employees. Many physiological burdens are associated with the use of certain types of respirators. The weight of the respirator, breathing resistances during both normal operation and operation when the air-purifying element is overloaded, and rebreathing exhaled air from respirator "dead space" all can increase the physiologic burden of respirator use. Job and workplace conditions, such as the length of time a respirator must be worn, the level of physical exertion required of a respirator user, and environmental conditions, also can affect the physiological burden. In addition, workers who wear glasses or hearing aids may have problems achieving appropriate fit with some respirator facepieces.

Examples of respirator hazards include the following:

- An employee's health may be jeopardized by the wearing of a respirator (e.g., a cardiac/pulmonary disorder could be aggravated by respirator use)
- The wearing of a dirty respirator may cause dermatitis or ingestion of a hazardous chemical
- The sharing of a respirator may lead to transmittal of disease

Respirators for IDLH atmospheres

Some atmospheric conditions could pose an immediate threat to life, cause irreversible adverse health effects, or impair an individual's ability to escape. The standard requires employers to provide the following respirators for employee use in such IDLH atmospheres:

- A full facepiece pressure-demand SCBA certified by NIOSH for a minimum service life of 30 minutes
- A combination full facepiece pressure-demand supplied-air respirator with auxiliary self-contained air supply

Respirators provided only for escape from IDLH atmospheres must be NIOSH-certified for escape from the atmosphere in which they will be used. All oxygen-deficient atmospheres must be considered IDLH.

If the employer demonstrates that, under all foreseeable conditions, the oxygen concentration can be maintained within specified ranges, then any atmosphere-supplying respirator may be used.

Procedures for IDLH atmospheres

For all IDLH atmospheres, the employer must ensure that

- one employee or, when needed, more than one employee is located outside the IDLH atmosphere
- visual, voice, or signal line communication is maintained between employees in the IDLH atmosphere
- employees located outside the IDLH atmosphere are trained and equipped to provide effective emergency rescue
- the employer or designee is notified before employees located outside the IDLH atmosphere enter the IDLH atmosphere to provide emergency rescue
- the employer or designee authorized to do so by the employer, once notified, provides necessary assistance appropriate to the situation
- employees located outside IDLH atmospheres are equipped with pressure-demand or other positive-pressure SCBAs, or a pressure-demand or other positive-pressure supplied-air respirator with auxiliary SCBA, and either appropriate retrieval equipment for removing employees who enter the hazardous atmospheres or equivalent means for rescue where retrieval equipment is not required

According to OSHA guidance, planning is critical for effective response to emergency situations through the development of specific emergency procedures. The procedures should address how the employer will be notified when standby personnel enter the IDLH atmosphere to provide emergency rescue and what actions will be taken or what forms of assistance will be provided by the employer. Emergency procedures must be developed and included in the employer's written respirator program.

Voice, radio, or signal line are permitted for work performed outside of visual contact. Communication protocols must be established that allow the standby person to monitor who is inside to alert entrants if evacuation becomes necessary. It is not sufficient to rely on the employees in the IDLH area to call for help when needed.

OSHA notes that in facilities where an uncontrolled release of a hazardous substance could create an emergency IDLH atmosphere, employers must follow the requirements of the HAZWOPER standard 29 CFR 1910.120.

Procedures for interior structural firefighting

OSHA has defined "interior structural firefighting" to mean the physical activity of fire suppression, rescue, or both inside buildings or enclosed structures that are beyond the incipient stage. This includes firefighting to control or extinguish a fire that is in an advanced stage of burning, or is producing large amounts of smoke, heat, and toxic products of combustion. Firefighter exposure during this activity is extremely hazardous. The atmosphere is considered IDLH, and the use of SCBA is required.

By contrast, incipient-stage firefighting involves the control or extinguishment of a fire in the initial or beginning stage using portable fire extinguishers or small hose lines without the need for PPE. It is the incident commander's responsibility, based on training and experience, to judge whether a fire is an interior structural fire and how it will be attacked.

In interior structural fires, the respiratory-protection standard requires that

- at least two employees enter the IDLH atmosphere and remain in visual or voice contact with one another
- at least two employees are located outside the IDLH atmosphere at all times
- all employees engaged in interior structural firefighting use SCBAs

One of the two individuals located outside the IDLH atmosphere may be assigned to an additional role, such as safety officer or incident commander in charge of the emergency, as long as the individual is able to perform assistance or rescue activities without jeopardizing the safety or health of any firefighter working at the site.

OSHA notes that nothing in this requirement is meant to preclude firefighters from performing emergency rescue activities before an entire team has assembled.

According to OSHA's inspection procedures, the two firefighters stationed outside during interior structural firefighting must be trained, equipped, and prepared to enter if necessary to rescue the firefighters inside. However, the incident commander has the responsibility and flexibility to determine when more than two outside firefighters are necessary given the circumstances of the fire. The agency clarifies that the "two-in/two-out" rule does not require an arithmetic progression for every firefighter inside (i.e., the rule should not be interpreted as four-in/four-out, eight-in/eight-out, etc.).

Electronic methods of communication, such as radios, must not be substituted for direct visual contact between the team members in the danger area. However, OSHA clarifies that reliable electronic communication devices are not prohibited under the standard and have value in augmenting communication. Such devices may be used to communicate between inside team members and outside standby personnel.

Respirators for atmospheres that are not IDLH

The employer must provide a respirator that is adequate to protect the health of the employee and ensure compliance with all other OSHA statutory and regulatory requirements, under routine and reasonably foreseeable emergency situations. The respirator selected must be appropriate for the chemical state and physical form of the contaminant. For protection against gases and vapors, the employer must provide either of the following:

- An atmosphere-supplying respirator
- An air-purifying respirator, provided that the respirator is equipped with an ESLI certified by NIOSH for the contaminant; or, if there is no ESLI appropriate for conditions in the employer's workplace, the employer creates a change schedule for canisters and cartridges based on objective information or data that will ensure that canisters and cartridges are changed before the end of their service life

For protection against particulates, the employer must provide one of the following:

- An atmosphere-supplying respirator
- An air-purifying respirator equipped with a filter certified by NIOSH under 30 CFR 11 as a HEPA filter, or an air-purifying respirator equipped with a filter certified for particulates by NIOSH under 42 CFR 84

For contaminants that consist primarily of particles with mass median aerodynamic diameters of at least 2 micrometers, an air-purifying respirator equipped with any filter certified for particulates by NIOSH is allowed.

Medical evaluation

Using a respirator may place on employees a physiological burden that varies with the type of respirator worn, the job and workplace conditions in which the respirator is used, and the medical status of the employee. The employer must provide a medical evaluation to determine the employee's ability to use a respirator before the employee is fit tested or required to use the respirator in the workplace. The employer may discontinue an employee's medical evaluations when the employee is no longer required to use a respirator.

Additional medical evaluations

At a minimum, the employer must provide additional medical evaluations if

- an employee reports medical signs or symptoms that are related to ability to use a respirator
- a physician or other licensed healthcare professional, supervisor, or the respirator-program administrator informs the employer that an employee needs to be reevaluated
- information from the respiratory protection program, including observations made during fit testing and program evaluation, indicates a need for employee reevaluation
- a change occurs in workplace conditions (e.g., physical work effort, protective clothing, temperature) that may result in a substantial increase in the physiological burden placed on an employee

Medical evaluations are required for all respirator users except for employees who voluntarily use dust masks and for those who would use escape-only respirators. SCBAs are not considered escape-only respirators. Employees who refuse to be medically evaluated cannot be assigned to work in areas where they are required to wear a respirator.

Fit testing

Before an employee may be required to use any respirator with a negative- or positive-pressure tight-fitting facepiece, the employee must be fit tested with the same make, model, style, and size of respirator that will be used.

Employees who use tight-fitting facepiece respirators must pass an appropriate qualitative fit test (QLFT) or quantitative fit test (QNFT). The employer must ensure that an employee using a tight-fitting facepiece respirator is fit tested prior to initial use of the respirator; whenever using a respirator facepiece different in size, style, model, or make; or and at least annually thereafter.

A fit test is not required for voluntary users or for escape-only respirators.

Qualitative fit testing may be used to fit test negative-pressure air-purifying respirators if they will only be used in atmospheres less than 10 times the PEL. For greater concentrations, QLFT must be used.

An additional fit test must be conducted whenever the employee reports—or the employer, physician, or other licensed healthcare professional, supervisor, or program administrator makes visual observations of—changes in the employee's physical condition that could affect respirator fit. Such conditions include, but are not limited to, facial scarring, dental changes, cosmetic surgery, or obvious change in body weight.

If after passing a QLFT or QNFT the employee subsequently notifies the employer, program administrator, supervisor, physician, or other licensed healthcare professional that the fit of the respirator is unacceptable, the employee must be given a reasonable opportunity to select a different respirator facepiece and be retested.

The fit test must be administered using OSHA-accepted QLFT or QNFT protocol. The OSHA-accepted QLFT and QNFT protocols and procedures are contained in Appendix A of 29 CFR 1910.134.

Facepiece seal protection

The employer must not permit respirators with tight-fitting facepieces to be worn by employees who have

- facial hair that either comes between the sealing surface of the facepiece and the face or that interferes with valve function

- any condition that interferes with the face-to-facepiece seal or valve function

For all tight-fitting respirators, the employer must ensure that employees perform a user seal check each time they put on the respirator.

Corrective lenses

When corrective lenses must be worn as part of the respirator facepiece, the facepiece and lenses should be fitted by a qualified individual and provide good vision, comfort, and a gas-tight seal. Wearing of contact lenses in a contaminated atmosphere with a respirator may not be allowed. If corrective spectacles or goggles are required, they must be worn so as not to affect the facepiece fit.

Continuing respirator effectiveness

Maintain appropriate surveillance of work-area conditions and degree of employee exposure or stress. When there is a change in work-area conditions or degree of employee exposure or stress that may affect respirator effectiveness, the employer must reevaluate the continued effectiveness of the respirator.

The surveillance procedures may include continuous or periodic monitoring, on-site observations, and notation of problems. The intensity of the surveillance should be tailored to the hazards present in the workplace. Highly hazardous substances that pose acute respiratory hazards merit a higher degree of surveillance.

The employer must ensure that employees leave the respirator-use area

- to wash their faces and respirator facepieces as necessary to prevent eye or skin irritation associated with respirator use
- if they detect vapor or gas breakthrough, changes in breathing resistance, or leakage of the facepiece
- to replace the respirator or the filter, cartridge, or canister elements

If the employee detects vapor or gas breakthrough, changes in breathing resistance, or leakage of the facepiece, the employer must replace or repair the respirator before allowing the employee to return to the work area.

Maintenance and care

Employers must provide for the cleaning, disinfecting, storage, inspection, and repair of respirators used by employees.

Cleaning and disinfecting

Each respirator user must be provided with a respirator that is clean, sanitary, and in good working order. The employer must ensure that respirators are cleaned and disinfected as often as necessary to keep them in a sanitary condition.

To ensure that respirators are clean and in good working order, the employer may have respirators cleaned and repaired in a centralized operation where respirators are passed out to employees, or the employer may require the respirator user to perform all cleaning and respirator-maintenance functions.

Respirators issued to more than one employee must be cleaned and disinfected before being worn by another user. Individually wrapped cleaning towelettes may be used as an interim method in the cleaning schedule for individually assigned respirators, but they must not be the only method in place. During fit testing, towelettes also may be used among employees being tested; however, these respirators must be thoroughly cleaned at the end of each day.

Storage

All respirators must be stored to protect against damage, contamination, dust, sunlight, extreme temperatures, excessive moisture, and damaging chemicals, and they must be packed or stored to prevent deformation of the facepiece and exhalation valve.

Emergency-use respirators must be kept accessible to the work area, stored in compartments or in covers that are clearly marked as containing emergency respirators, and stored in accordance with any applicable manufacturer instructions.

Inspection

All respirators used in routine situations must be inspected before each use and during cleaning. All respirators maintained for use in emergency situations must be inspected at least monthly and in accordance with the manufacturer's recommendations, and they must be checked for proper function before and after each use.

SCBAs must be inspected monthly. Air and oxygen cylinders must be maintained in a fully charged state and must be recharged when the pressure falls to 90% of the manufacturer's recommended pressure level. The employer must determine that the regulator and warning devices function properly.

Emergency escape-only respirators carried by employees must be inspected before being taken into the workplace for potential use.

Do the following with respirators maintained for emergency use:

- Certify the respirator by documenting the date on which the inspection was performed, the name (or signature) of the person who made the inspection, the findings, the required remedial action, and a serial number or other means of identifying the inspected respirator.

- Provide this information on a tag or label that is attached to the storage compartment for the respirator, is kept with the respirator, or is included in inspection reports stored as paper or electronic files. This information must be maintained until replaced following a subsequent certification.

Repairs

Respirators that fail an inspection or are otherwise found to be defective must be removed from service and discarded, repaired, or adjusted. A respirator is defective if one or more of its components is missing, damaged, or visibly deteriorated.

An appropriately trained person must be responsible for performing repairs or adjustments to respirators. An employer who does not keep on hand sufficient parts to allow respirators to be repaired will need to remove those respirators from service until suitable repairs can be made.

Only the respirator manufacturer's NIOSH-approved parts designed for the particular respirator being repaired can be used to repair a respirator.

The employer must develop some means of ensuring that defective respirators are not used in the workplace. The employer can comply by placing an out-of-service tag on the respirator or by removing the respirator from the work area.

Breathing-air quality and use

Employers are required to provide employees using atmosphere-supplying respirators (supplied-air and SCBA) with breathing gases of high purity. Compressed air, compressed oxygen, liquid air, and liquid oxygen used for respiration must meet required specifications.

Identification of filters, cartridges, and canisters

The employer must ensure that all filters, cartridges, and canisters used in the workplace are labeled and color-coded with the NIOSH-approval label, and they must ensure the label is not removed and remains legible.

Training

Supervisors and workers must be properly instructed in the selection, use, and maintenance of respirators. Instruction must be conducted by competent individuals.

Employers are required to provide effective training to employees who are required to use respirators. The training must be comprehensive, understandable, and annual (or more often, if necessary).

The employer must ensure that each employee can demonstrate knowledge of at least the following:

- Why the respirator is necessary and how improper fit, usage, or maintenance can compromise the protective effect of the respirator
- What the limitations and capabilities of the respirator are
- How to use the respirator effectively in emergency situations, including situations in which the respirator malfunctions
- How to inspect, put on and remove, use, and check the seals of the respirator
- What the procedures are for maintenance and storage of the respirator
- How to recognize medical signs and symptoms that may limit or prevent effective respirator use
- The general requirements of the respiratory-protection standard

Training should provide employees an opportunity to handle the respirator, have it fitted properly, test its facepiece-to-face seal, wear it in normal air to become familiar with it, and wear it in a test atmosphere.

Every wearer must receive fitting instructions that include demonstration and practice in how the respirator should be worn, how to adjust it, and how to determine whether it fits properly.

Retraining must be administered annually and when the following situations occur:

- Changes in the workplace or type of respirator render previous training obsolete
- Inadequacies in the employee's knowledge or use of the respirator indicate that the employee has not retained the requisite understanding or skill
- Any other situation arises in which retraining appears necessary to ensure safe respirator use

Program evaluation

The respiratory-protection standard requires employers to conduct evaluations of the workplace to ensure that the written respiratory-protection program is being carried out properly.

Employers must observe and consult employees to determine whether they have any problems with the program and to ensure that the respirators are used properly.

Any problems that are identified during this assessment must be corrected. Factors to be assessed include, but are not limited to, the following:

- Respirator fit (including the ability to use the respirator without interfering with effective workplace performance)
- Appropriate respirator selection for the hazards to which the employee is exposed
- Proper respirator use under the workplace conditions the employee encounters
- Proper respirator maintenance

Recordkeeping

Employers must establish and retain written information regarding medical evaluations, fit testing, and the respirator program. This information will facilitate employee involvement in the respirator program, help the employer audit the adequacy of the program, and provide a record for compliance determinations by OSHA.

Medical evaluation

Records of required medical evaluations must be retained and made available in accordance with OSHA's standard for access to employee exposure and medical records under 29 CFR 1910.1020.

The record of the medical evaluation must include the result of the medical questionnaire and, if applicable, a copy of the physician or other licensed healthcare professional's written opinion and recommendations, including the results of relevant medical examinations and tests.

Fit test records

The employer must establish a record of the QLFT and QNFT administered to an employee, including the following:

- The name or identification of the employee tested
- Type of fit test performed
    - Specific make, model, style, and size of respirator tested
    - Date of test
    - The pass/fail results for QLFTs or the fit factor and strip chart recording or other recording of the test results for QNFTs

Fit test records must be retained for respirator users until the next fit test is administered.

Written program

In addition to medical evaluation and fit test records, a written copy of the current respirator program must be retained by the employer. All written materials required to be retained must be made available upon request to affected employees and to OSHA for examination and copying.

Welding (1910.254 and 252)

at a glance

The welding standard covers hazards from welding that involve certain alloys and compounds such as zinc, lead, cadmium, or mercury. Ventilation, eye protection, flameproof screens, and fire watches are also addressed.

Arc-welding cables with damaged insulation or exposed, bare conductors shall be replaced (29 CFR 1910.254[d][9][iii]).

Refer to 29 CFR 1910.252(c)(5) through (10) for special considerations when welding operations require fluxes, coverings, coatings, or alloys that involve fluorine compounds, zinc, lead, beryllium, cadmium, or mercury.

Mechanical ventilation must be provided when

- welding or cutting in a space where there is less than 10,000 cubic feet per welder
- the overhead height is less than 16 feet (29 CFR 1910.252[c][2][i][A] and [B])

Proper shielding and eye protection to prevent exposure of personnel from welding hazards must be provided (29 CFR 1910.252[b][2][i][B] through [D] and [F] through [H]).

Workers or other persons adjacent to the welding areas shall be protected from the welding rays by noncombustible or flameproof screens or shields or shall be required to wear appropriate goggles. The screens shall be so arranged that no serious restriction of ventilation exists (29 CFR 1910.252[b][2][iii] and 1910[c][1][iii]).

Proper precautions (isolating welding and cutting, removing fire hazards and combustibles, and providing a fire watch) for fire prevention must be taken in areas where welding or other "hot work" is being done (29 CFR 1910.252[a]).

Welding in confined spaces

All welding and cutting operations that are performed in confined spaces (such as a tank, boiler, or pressure vessel) must be adequately ventilated to prevent the accumulation of toxic materials or possible oxygen deficiency (29 CFR 1910.252[c][4]).

In such circumstances where it is impossible to provide such ventilation, airline respirators or hose masks approved by NIOSH for this purpose must be used (29 CFR 1910.252[c][4][ii]).

In areas immediately hazardous to life, airline respirators with escape air bottles or SCBA must be used. The breathing equipment must be approved by NIOSH (29 CFR 1910.252[c][4][iii]).

Where welding operations are carried on in confined spaces and where welders and helpers are provided with airline respirators or SCBA, a worker must be stationed on the outside of such confined spaces to ensure the safety of those working within (29 CFR 1910.252[c][4][iv] and 1910.146[d][6]). Oxygen must never be used for ventilation (29 CFR 1910.252[c][4][v]).

Workplace violence (voluntary guideline)

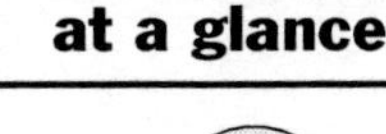

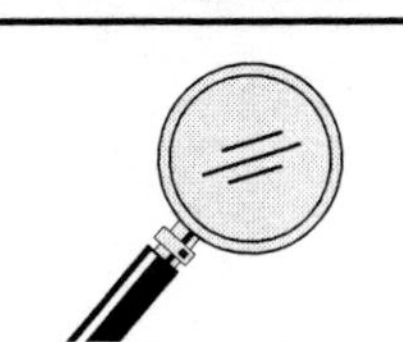

OSHA has released guidelines for preventing workplace violence in healthcare settings. It can also cite workplace hazards under its general duty clause.

OSHA identifies violence in the workplace as a serious safety and health issue and recognizes that healthcare workers face a greater risk of job-related violence than do members of the general workforce.

Even though OSHA does not have standards that specifically address workplace violence, it has published ***Guidelines for Preventing Workplace Violence for Health Care and Social Service Workers*** (2004), which provides recommendations for reducing workplace violence.

The agency encourages employers to establish violence prevention programs for all healthcare facilities and recommends a written plan for businesses with more than 10 employees.

OSHA guidelines

According to the guidelines, a workplace violence prevention program should accomplish the following:

- Create a clear policy of zero tolerance for workplace violence, verbal and nonverbal threats, and related actions
- Ensure that managers, supervisors, coworkers, clients, patients, and visitors know about this policy
- Ensure that no employee who reports or experiences workplace violence faces reprisals
- Encourage prompt incident reports and timely suggestions to reduce risks

- Require records of incidents to assess risk and measure progress
- Outline a comprehensive plan for maintaining security in the workplace
- Assign responsibility and authority for the program
- Ensure that adequate resources are available
- Affirm management commitment to a worker-supportive environment
- Set up a company briefing as part of the initial effort to address issues

The guidelines identify six components of any effective safety and health program for preventing workplace violence:

- Management commitment and employee involvement
- Work-site analysis
- Hazard prevention and control
- Safety and health training
- Recordkeeping
- Program evaluation

Management commitment and employee involvement

Management should provide the resources to deal effectively with workplace violence and assign responsibility for the program administration. Managers, supervisors, and employees should understand their obligations and accept accountability. Employees should report violent incidents promptly and accurately.

Management's commitment includes evaluating the components of a successful workplace violence program annually as a reflection of the organization's culture and as a function of providing accessibility and resources for staff. As much as preventing episodes of workplace violence, how an organization manages actual events, including follow-up, is often the "test" for employees.

Work-site analysis

A work-site analysis is a common sense, detailed examination of the facility to identify existing or potential hazards for workplace violence. It should address procedures, operations, and environmental risk factors. The analysis could proceed from the work of management-and-employee teams, such as a threat-assessment team, or a patient-assault team.

This process complements prudent risk-management strategies and should receive an annual review. An additional review should occur whenever changes in the care provided or the environment suggest a "mid-course correction."

The recommended program for work-site analysis includes, but is not limited to

- analyzing and tracking records
- screening surveys
- analyzing workplace security

Hazard prevention and control

After identifying hazards from a work-site analysis, establish control measures through administrative, engineering, and work practice controls to minimize and prevent hazards.

Administrative and work-practice controls may include

- incident reporting
- use of a trained response team for emergencies and trained security officers to deal with aggressive behavior
- restricted-access procedures
- adequate staffing
- use of the buddy system

Engineering controls may include

- alarm systems
- access control systems
- panic buttons
- metal detectors
- closed-circuit television
- other security devices selected and used based on the hazards present

Postincident response

The manner in which the employer responds to workplace violence is an essential part of prevention and control.

Workplace violence prevention programs should provide comprehensive treatment for victimized employees and employees traumatized by witnessing workplace violence. A comprehensive plan provides for prompt medical treatment and psychological evaluation whenever an assault takes place, regardless of its severity. The plan should accommodate transportation to an off-site medical facility.

Recognize that victims of workplace violence suffer a variety of consequences in addition to their actual physical injuries. These consequences may include psychological trauma, fear of returning to work, and heightened sensitivity to criticism by supervisors or managers.

Follow-up programs will help employees deal with problems and help prepare them to confront or prevent future incidents.

Safety and health training

Training and education heighten staff awareness of potential security hazards and how to take measures to protect themselves and coworkers. Every employee should understand the concept of "universal precautions for violence"—violence should always be considered a very real possibility but one that is avoidable or can be mitigated through preparation.

Employees facing safety and security hazards should receive formal training on the specific hazards associated with the job duties, including instructions to limit physical interventions in workplace altercations whenever possible, unless enough staff or emergency response teams and security personnel are available.

New and reassigned employees should receive hazard-specific orientation before their first independent assignment.

Ongoing education programs should include annual refreshers and frequent update sessions, especially in larger organizations where it is difficult to reach all workers. Additionally, depending on job functions, basic competency expectations might be part of the education program. For instance, security officers, or even clinical staff with the likelihood of risky interactions, would probably benefit from ongoing competency assessment.

Recordkeeping

Keeping records of the activities and events of the violence prevention program will help identify deficiencies in the program and provide invaluable data for evaluation. Also, it will help create a climate within the organization that encourages reporting of all events concerning violent behavior. Good records help employers determine the severity of the problem, evaluate methods of hazard control, and identify training needs.

Types of records include the following:

- OSHA log of work-related injury and illness (OSHA form 300).
- Medical reports of work injury and supervisors' reports for each recorded assault.
- Records of incidents of abuse, verbal attacks, or aggressive behavior that may be threatening, such as pushing or shouting, and acts of aggression toward other clients. This record may be kept as part of an assault incident report.

- Information on patients with a history of past violence, drug abuse, or criminal activity recorded on the patient's chart.
- Documentation of minutes of safety meetings, records of hazard analyses, and corrective actions recommended and taken.
- Records of all training programs, attendees, and qualifications of trainers.

Program evaluation

As part of the comprehensive workplace violence prevention program, employers should conduct regular evaluations of safety and security measures. Evaluations should occur at least annually and whenever an incident occurs, as a component investigation follow-up. The evaluation should include participation from senior management and employees closest to the care environment, including managers, supervisors, and frontline employees.

Regular input from managers, supervisors, and frontline staff enhances the organization's ability to identify deficiencies and implement meaningful corrective actions quickly.

Any evaluation of the violence prevention program is virtually useless without appropriate and timely communication throughout the organization. Deficiencies will remain if staff are not invested in the improvement process, and that investment is most unlikely in the absence of good communication.

Use meetings, newsletters, posters, and surveys to communicate the importance of a climate of safety. If employees do not feel safe, they may not proactively manage or participate in the workplace violence prevention program. Dialogue is the key to success in managing the safety and security of the organization.

Xylene

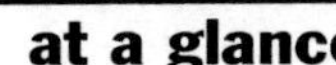

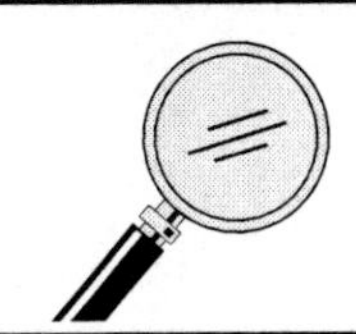

Xylene is regulated under OSHA's air-contaminants standard 1910.1000 through PELs.

Xylene

Xylene, also known as xylol or dimethylbenzene, is an aromatic organic compound used as a solvent in clinical laboratories, such as histology or pathology labs, as well as in industrial processes and for common industrial and consumer products such as paint, gasoline, and cleaning fluids.

Xylene is a clear, colorless, sweet-smelling liquid that is flammable, readily evaporates at room temperature, does not mix well with water, and mixes with alcohol and many other chemicals. It can be detected by odor at a level of approximately 0.08 ppm–3.7 ppm and can be tasted in water beginning at 0.53 ppm–1.8 ppm.

In clinical labs, xylene is used to remove ethyl alcohol and paraffin from cassettes for tissue processing and slide-staining procedures. It also is commonly used in oil-immersion microscopy.

Employees at highest risk of exposure in clinical or healthcare settings include biomedical-laboratory workers, who may be exposed to high indoor levels of xylene, especially in buildings with poor ventilation. Employees also may be exposed through skin contact with products containing xylene. Small amounts of benzene, naphthalene, toluene, and other benzene derivatives also are found in preparations of xylene used in oil-immersion microscopy in mycobacterium and cytology laboratories.

Forms of xylene

There are three forms, or isomers, of xylene: meta-, ortho-, and para-xylene. The term "total xylenes" refers to all three forms of xylene as well as mixed xylene, which contains all three isomers and also usually contains 6%–15% ethylbenzene. Mixed xylene typically is used in clinical laboratories, while in commercial preparations, the meta-xylene isomer predominates. Xylene is registered under Chemical Abstracts Service (CAS) No. 1330–20–7.

Toxicology

Xylene typically enters the body through inhalation, skin contact, or ingestion of contaminated food or water. Xylene vapors are absorbed rapidly by the lungs, which retain 50%–75% of inhaled vapors. Physical exercise increases absorption.

Some xylene may be exhaled unchanged, but most is broken down to other chemicals in the liver and lungs. Breakdown products are rapidly excreted, mainly in urine, beginning as soon as two hours after breathing contaminated air. The body usually clears most xylene within 18 hours of exposure, although its storage in fat or muscle may prolong clearance time.

Adverse health effects

Dose, duration, and route of exposure to xylene will determine whether adverse health effects will occur and what the type and severity of those effects will be. Other chemical exposures as well as individual characteristics such as chemical sensitivity, age, gender, nutritional status, family traits, lifestyle, and health status also determine adverse effects.

Acute

Short-term high-level exposures can cause irritation of the skin, eyes, nose, and throat; breathing difficulty; impaired lung function; delayed response to visual stimulus; impaired memory; stomach discomfort; and possible changes in the liver and kidneys.

Both short- and long-term exposure to high concentrations of xylene also can affect the nervous system, bringing on headaches, lack of muscle coordination, dizziness, confusion, and changes in sense of balance. Exposure to very high levels of xylene for even a short period of time can cause death.

Chronic

Long-term effects of xylene exposure still are unclear, but some researchers believe that such exposure can impair the immune system. It is also thought that xylene can sensitize the myocardium to endogenous hormones such as epinephrine, possibly causing severe myocardial arrhythmias. Currently, there is no evidence that xylene exposure affects any blood components or blood-forming tissues.

Long-term xylene exposure has been studied mainly among workers in industries that make or use xylene, and many of the health effects may have been caused by exposure to other airborne chemicals.

Several studies of occupational data conclude that months or years of exposure to high levels of xylene or other organic solvents can cause possibly irreversible changes to the central nervous system, manifested by symptoms of general weakness, headache, irritability, sleeplessness, loss of memory, and tinnitus (ringing in the ears). Long-term inhalation exposure to high levels of xylene vapors has been shown to cause reversible neuropsychiatric disturbances and other behavioral changes. Healthcare workers exposed over a number of years to vapors from xylene and other organic solvents also showed a higher incidence of chronic bronchitis and other respiratory problems.

Reproductive effects

Exposure of pregnant women to high levels of xylene may cause harmful effects to the fetus. Animal studies indicate that high exposures may cause increased numbers of fetal deaths, decreased weight, skeletal changes, and delayed skeletal development.

The mother's health also may be at stake. Increased menstrual disorders, infertility, and certain pathological pregnancy conditions, such as miscarriage and hemorrhage during delivery, have been linked to chronic xylene exposure.

Carcinogenicity

Neither the IARC nor the EPA has found adequate information from animal studies to determine that xylene is carcinogenic. But both the IARC and EPA have determined that xylene is a toxic substance that may have the potential to be carcinogenic to humans.

A study of workers who were exposed to xylene vapor over many years indicates that xylene may be involved in the development of lymphocytic leukemia; however, because other solvents were present in the inhaled vapors, the data cannot be used to label xylene as a potential carcinogen.

The EPA, using the guidelines of the Carcinogen Assessment Group, has labeled xylene a Group D substance, defined as unclassifiable as to potential to cause cancer in humans.

Exposure limits

OSHA and the ACGIH recommend that the TWA-TLV of xylene be established at 100 ppm (435 mg/m^3).

OSHA's air-contaminants standard sets an occupational PEL of 100 ppm of xylene in air averaged over an eight-hour work day, and a STEL of 150 ppm (655 mg/m^3) over 15 minutes. Both limits are enforceable by law.

NIOSH has recommended an exposure limit of 100 ppm of xylene averaged over a workday up to 10 hours long in a 40-hour work week. NIOSH also has recommended that exposure to xylene not exceed 150 ppm for longer than 15 minutes or a ceiling limit of 200 ppm over 10 minutes. NIOSH has classified xylene exposures of 10,000 ppm as IDLH.

Work practices

Generally, xylene exposures in histology and pathology laboratories occur because

- most tissue-processing procedures are done in the general work area, not in designated laboratory exhaust hoods.
- workers lack, or are unwilling to use, specially designated, isolated, and well-ventilated areas for procedures involving xylene or other hazardous chemicals.
- xylene solutions used in special stains and tissue processing are dumped down drains without flushing the sink and drain with running water. Spent xylene should not be disposed of in any way not authorized by the EPA, state agencies, or local water-quality authorities.
- fume-hood charcoal filters are not periodically replaced, serviced, or maintained.
- fume-hood fans often are not activated during hazardous procedures.
- protective gloves often are not worn because many technicians consider them too clumsy.
- slide holders often are removed from xylene solutions without using forceps and with unprotected hands, and slides coated with xylene typically are handled without gloves.
- no respiratory protection is used during xylene-solution dumping.
- lab coats or aprons that are wet from xylene splashes are not changed.
- xylene containers are stored with loose lids.
- paper towels used to soak up xylene spills are disposed of improperly—for example, in a wastebasket—allowing evaporation into ambient air and potential exposure.

Even the most stringent threshold standards and diligent monitoring will not prevent exposures from occurring in the laboratory if the employer does not install and maintain adequate engineering controls and safety equipment (including respirators), provide proper employee training on the equipment, institute mandatory safe-laboratory procedures, and designate special areas for the use of hazardous chemicals. Employees also must fully cooperate and use equipment and controls properly and regularly.

Medical surveillance

The preemployment medical examination is a primary component in protecting employees from exposure to xylene vapors. Employees should be examined for preexisting conditions that could place them at higher risk of developing xylene-related symptoms.

Medical surveillance, which includes a complete physical examination and appropriate laboratory diagnostic tests, should be instituted if workers show signs or symptoms of xylene poisoning or if exposure to high levels of xylene is suspected. The medical examination should include

- skin examination for xylene toxicity
- liver function tests and urinalysis
- neurological testing for disorders of the central nervous system

Medical surveillance will establish a baseline for future environmental exposure monitoring. Available tests can indicate only exposure to xylene; they cannot be used to predict which health effects, if any, will develop.

Environmental monitoring

Monitoring the laboratory environment for xylene contamination is critical if high-level xylene exposure is suspected (e.g., through container breakage) or if employees develop signs or symptoms of xylene exposure. By determining airborne xylene vapor concentrations, it is possible to establish or refute the presence of overexposure and correlation to worker signs and symptoms.

Personal monitoring is done using badge-type organic-vapor monitors. Periodically, a sampling train is used for active sampling of general environmental air. OSHA does not specify an approved monitoring method. NIOSH Method 1501—Aromatic Hydrocarbons—is recognized by industrial hygiene practitioners as the best available method.

It is advisable to contract with a qualified industrial hygienist to perform the monitoring to ensure actual "breathing-zone" exposure levels. Industrial hygienists also will typically recommend engineering, administrative, and personal protective controls to reduce or eliminate hazardous vapor concentrations.

If complaints persist even after air monitoring shows that xylene levels are in compliance with the PELs or TWAs, a health evaluation of the employees may be advisable. Contact the local OSHA office for advice.

Xylene substitution

Certain solvent products based on a citrus extract called d-limonene, referred to as "orange oil" (CAS No. 5989–27–5), have proven to be a less irritating xylene substitute for tissue fixation. Limonene also is used in commercial solvents and degreasers.

Clinical laboratories that wish to try limonene-based products should be aware that orange oil is a potent defatting agent that can cause severe skin and eye irritation. Limonene, whose chemical name is 4-isopropenyl-1-methylcyclohexene, is a skin irritant and sensitizer. Limonene is not regulated by OSHA or any other standard-setting organization.

Xylene disposal and recycling

Under the RCRA, the generator of xylene waste is responsible for its proper disposal. Regulations under the law permit laboratories to either recycle xylene or have it transported to an EPA-licensed hazardous-waste-disposal facility. Disposal costs, however, are increasing as the number of dumping sites decreases and licensing for disposal facilities becomes more difficult.

As an alternative, solvent-recycling devices can recover up to 80% of the xylene and achieve nearly 99% purity. Through a distillation process, xylene is boiled off from contaminants and recovered by vapor condensation. Material and disposal costs are greatly reduced by recycling, although properly trained equipment operations personnel are needed. Xylene recycling is usually only cost- and labor-effective in larger facilities that produce a high volume of waste xylene.

Appendix A: State occupational safety and health plans

explanation

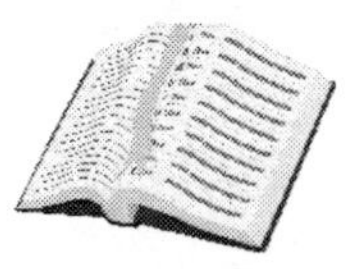

Section 18 of the Occupational Safety and Health Act of 1970 encourages states to develop and operate their own job safety and health programs. Federal OSHA is responsible for approving and monitoring state plans.

Twenty-six states operate OSHA-approved state plans and have adopted their own standards and enforcement policies. Plans in Connecticut, New Jersey, New York, and the Virgin Islands cover public sector (i.e., state and local government) employment only.

For the most part, the state plans standards are identical to federal OSHA. Some states, however, have adopted different standards applicable to the healthcare industry or may have different enforcement policies. For example, parts of California's bloodborne pathogen standard are more rigorous than the federal standard.

If your facility operates in a state with its own occupational safety and health plan, check the Web sites or call the state-plan offices listed below for regulations different from federal OSHA. A list of state plans with contact information and links is also available at *www.osha.gov*.

States with approved occupational safety and health plans

Alaska

Alaska Department of Labor and Workforce Development

P.O. Box 21149

1111 W. 8th Street, Room 306

Juneau, AK 99802-1149

Greg O'Claray, commissioner

(907) 465-2700/Fax: (907) 465-2784

Grey Mitchell, Director

(907) 465-4855/Fax: (907) 465-6012

http://labor.state.ak.us/lss/home.htm

Arizona

Industrial Commission of Arizona

800 W. Washington

Phoenix, AZ 85007-2922

Larry Etchechury, director, ICA

(602) 542-4411/Fax: (602) 542-1614

Darin Perkins, program director

(602) 542-5795/Fax: (602) 542-1614

www.ica.state.az.us/ADOSH/oshatop.htm

California

California Department of Industrial Relations

455 Golden Gate Avenue, 10th Floor

San Francisco, CA 94102

John Rea, acting director

(415) 703-5050/Fax: (415) 703-5059

Len Welsh, chief, Cal/OSHA

(415) 703-5100/Fax: (415) 703-5114

Vicky Heza, deputy chief, Cal/OSHA

(714) 939-8093/Fax (714) 939-8094

www.dir.ca.gov/occupational_safety.html

Connecticut

Connecticut Department of Labor

200 Folly Brook Boulevard

Wethersfield, CT 06109

Shaun Cashman, commissioner

(860) 566-5123/Fax: (860) 566-1520

Conn-OSHA

38 Wolcott Hill Road

Wethersfield, CT 06109

Richard Palo, director

(860) 263-6900/Fax: (860) 263-6940

www.ctdol.state.ct.us/osha/osha.htm

Hawaii

Hawaii Department of Labor and Industrial Relations

830 Punchbowl Street

Honolulu, HI 96813

Nelson B. Befitel, director

(808) 586-8844/Fax: (808) 586-9099

Allan Yokoyama, acting administrator

(808) 586-9116/Fax: (808) 586-9104

http://hawaii.gov/labor/

Indiana

Indiana Department of Labor

State Office Building

402 West Washington Street, Room W195

Indianapolis, IN 46204-2751

Miguel Rivera, commissioner

(317) 232-2378/Fax: (317) 233-3790

Tim Crouse, acting deputy commissioner

(317) 232-3325/Fax: (317) 233-3790

www.in.gov/labor/iosha/index.html

Iowa

Iowa Division of Labor

1000 E. Grand Avenue

Des Moines, IA 50319-0209

Byron K. Orton, commissioner

(515) 281-6432/Fax: (515) 281-4698

Mary L. Bryant, administrator

(515) 242-5870/Fax: (515) 281-7995

www.iowaworkforce.org/labor/index.html

Kentucky

Kentucky Labor Cabinet

1047 U.S. Highway 127 South, Suite 4

Frankfort, KY 40601

Joe Norsworthy, secretary

(502) 564-3070/Fax: (502) 564-5387

William Ralston, federal\state coordinator

(502) 564-3070 ext.240/Fax: (502) 564-1682

www.labor.ky.gov/osh/index.htm

Maryland

Maryland Division of Labor and Industry

Department of Labor, Licensing and Regulation

1100 North Eutaw Street, Room 613

Baltimore, MD 21201-2206

Robert Lawson, commissioner

(410) 767-2241/Fax: (410) 767-2986

Jack English, acting assistant commissioner, MOSH

(410) 767-2190/Fax: (410) 333-7747

www.dllr.state.md.us/labor/mosh.html

Michigan

Michigan Department of Labor and Economic Growth

David C. Hollister, director

Michigan Occupational Safety and Health Administration

P.O. Box 30643

Lansing, MI 48909-8143

Doug Kalinowski, director

(517) 322-1814/Fax: (517) 322-1775

Martha Yoder, deputy director for enforcement

(517) 322-1817/Fax: (517) 322-1775

www.michigan.gov/cis/0,1607,7-154-11407---,00.html

Minnesota

Minnesota Department of Labor and Industry

443 Lafayette Road

St. Paul, MN 55155

Scott Brener, commissioner

(651) 284-5010 Fax: (651) 282-5405

Roslyn Wade, assistant commissioner

(651) 284-5371/Fax: (651) 282-2527

Patricia Todd, administrative director, OSHA Management Team

(651) 284-5372 Fax: (651) 297-2527

www.doli.state.mn.us/mnosha.html

Nevada

Nevada Division of Industrial Relations

400 West King Street, Suite 400

Carson City, NV 89703

Roger Bremmer, administrator

(775) 684-7260/Fax: (775) 687-6305

Occupational Safety and Health Enforcement Section

1301 N. Green Valley Parkway

Henderson, Nevada 89014

Tom Czehowski, chief administrative officer

(702) 486-9168/Fax: (702) 486-9020

[Las Vegas (702) 687-5240]

http://dirweb.state.nv.us/

New Jersey

New Jersey Department of Labor and Workforce Development

Office of Public Employees Occupational Safety & Health (PEOSH)

1 John Fitch Plaza

P.O. Box 386

Trenton, NJ 08625-0386

Thomas D. Carver, acting commissioner

(609) 292-2975/Fax: (609) 633-9271

Leonard Katz, assistant commissioner

(609) 292-2313/Fax: (609) 695-1314

Howard Black, director, PESOSH

(609) 292-0501/Fax: (609) 292-3749

Gary Ludwig, director, Occupational Health Service

(609) 984-1843/Fax: (609) 984-0849

www.state.nj.us/labor/lsse/lspeosh.html

New Mexico

New Mexico Environment Department

1190 St. Francis Drive, Suite 4050

P.O. Box 26110

Santa Fe, NM 87502

Ron Curry, Jr., secretary

(505) 827-2850/Fax: (505) 827-2836

Butch Tongate, chief

(505) 827-4230/Fax: (505) 827-4422

www.nmenv.state.nm.us/OHSB_website/ohsb_home.htm

New York

New York Department of Labor

New York Public Employee Safety and Health Program

State Office Campus Building 12, Room 158

Albany, NY 12240

Linda Angello, commissioner

(518) 457-2741/Fax: (518) 457-6908

Anthony Germano, director, Division of Safety and Health

(518) 457-3518/Fax: (518) 457-1519

Maureen Cox, program manager

(518) 457-1263/Fax: (518) 457-5545

www.labor.state.ny.us/workerprotection/safetyhealth/DOSH_PESH.shtm

North Carolina

North Carolina Department of Labor

4 West Edenton Street

Raleigh, NC 27601-1092

Cherie Berry, commissioner

(919) 733-0359/Fax: (919) 733-1092

Allen McNeely, deputy commissioner, OSH director

(919) 807-2861/Fax: (919) 807-2855

Kevin Beauregard, OSH assistant director

(919) 807-2863/Fax: (919) 807-2856

www.nclabor.com/osha/osh.htm

Oregon

Oregon Occupational Safety and Health Division

Department of Consumer and Business Services

350 Winter Street, NE, Room 430

Salem, OR 97301-3882

Michele Patterson, acting administrator

(503) 378-3272/Fax: (503) 947-7461

David Sparks, special assistant for Federal & External Affairs

(503) 378-3272/Fax: (503) 947-7461

www.orosha.org/

Puerto Rico

Puerto Rico Department of Labor

Prudencio Rivera Martínez Building

505 Muñoz Rivera Avenue

Hato Rey, PR 00918

Roman M. Velasco Gonzalez, secretary

(787) 754-2119/Fax: (787) 753-9550

José Droz-Alvarado, assistant secretary for Occupational Safety and Health

(787) 756-1100/(787) 754-2171/Fax: (787) 767-6051

www.osha.gov/oshdir/stateprogs/Puerto_Rico.html

South Carolina

South Carolina Department of Labor, Licensing, and Regulation

Koger Office Park, Kingstree Building

110 Centerview Drive

PO Box 11329

Columbia, SC 29211

Adrienne R. Youmans, director

(803) 896-4300/Fax: (803) 896-4393

Dottie Ison, administrator

(803) 896-7665/Fax: (803) 896-7670

Office of Voluntary Programs

(803) 896-7744/Fax: (803) 896-7750

www.llr.state.sc.us/osha.asp

Tennessee

Tennessee Department of Labor

710 James Robertson Parkway

Nashville, TN 37243-0659

James G. Neeley, commissioner
(615) 741-2582/Fax: (615) 741-5078
John Winkler, acting program director
(615) 741-2793/Fax: (615) 741-3325
www.state.tn.us/labor-wfd/

Utah

Utah Labor Commission
160 East 300 South, 3rd Floor
PO Box 146650
Salt Lake City, UT 84114-6650

R. Lee Ellertson, commissioner
(801) 530-6901/Fax: (801) 530-7906
Larry Patrick, administrator
(801) 530-6898/Fax: (801) 530-6390
www.uosh.utah.gov/

Vermont

Vermont Department of Labor
National Life Building – Drawer 20
Montpelier, VT 05620-3401

Patricia A. McDonald, commissioner
(802) 828-2288/Fax: (802) 828-2748
Robert McLeod, VOSHA compliance program manager
(802) 828-2765/Fax: (802) 828-2195
www.state.vt.us/labind/vosha.htm

Virgin Islands

Virgin Islands Department of Labor

3012 Golden Rock

Christiansted, St. Croix, Virgin Islands 00820-4660

Cecil R. Benjamin, commissioner

(340) 773-1994/Fax: (340) 773-1858

John Sheen, assistant commissioner

(340) 772-1315/Fax: (340) 772-4323

Francine Lang, program director

(340) 772-1315/Fax: (340) 772-4323

www.osha.gov/oshdir/stateprogs/Virgin_Islands.html

Virginia

Virginia Department of Labor and Industry

Powers-Taylor Building

13 South 13th Street

Richmond, VA 23219

C. Raymond Davenport, commissioner

(804) 786-2377/Fax: (804) 371-6524

Jay Withrow, director, Office of Legal Support

(804) 786-9873/Fax: (804) 786-8418

Glenn Cox, director, Safety Compliance, VOSHA

(804) 786-2391/Fax: (804) 371-6524

www.doli.state.va.us/index.html

Washington

Washington Department of Labor and Industries
General Administration Building
PO Box 44001
Olympia, WA 98504-4001

7273 Linderson Way SW
Tumwater, WA 98501-5414

Gary K. Weeks, director
(360) 902-4200/Fax: (360) 902-4202
Michael Wood, acting assistant director [PO Box 44600]
(360) 902-5495/Fax: (360) 902-5529
Steve Cant, program manager, Federal-State Operations [PO Box 44600]
(360) 902-5430/Fax: (360) 902-5529
www.lni.wa.gov/Safety/default.asp

Wyoming

Wyoming Department of Employment
Workers' Safety and Compensation Division
Cheyenne Business Center
1510 East Pershing Boulevard
Cheyenne, WY 82002

Gary W. Child, administrator
(307) 777-7700/Fax: (307) 777-5524
J.D. Danni, OSHA program manager
(307) 777-7786/Fax: (307) 777-3646
http://wydoe.state.wy.us/doe.asp?ID=7

Appendix B: OSHA standards training frequency

explanation

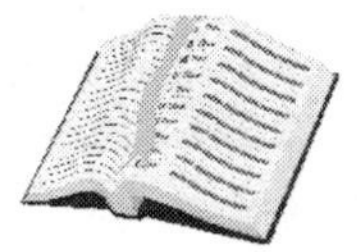

This table identifies training frequencies for OSHA standards for healthcare facilities. It includes only the standards in the OSHA Reference Guide that have specific training sections.

Standard	Applicability	Frequency
Asbestos General Industry 29 CFR 1910.1001	Employees exposed above the PELs; housekeeping employees who work in areas with ACM or PACM	Employees exposed above PELs: Upon assignment and annually thereafter; housekeeping employees: at least once per year
Asbestos Construction 29 CFR 1926.1101	Employees likely to be exposed above the PELs	Upon assignment and annually thereafter
Bloodborne Pathogens 29 CFR 1910.1030	All potentially exposed employees, including those in laundries or HIV/HBV laboratories and production facilities	Upon assignment to tasks where occupational exposure may occur and annually thereafter; also when duties or procedures change
Confined Spaces 29 CFR 1910.146	Employees entering confined spaces	Prior to first assignment of covered duties; prior to change in assigned duties; whenever a change in operations presents a new hazard; and whenever employee knowledge is inadequate
Emergency Plans 29 CFR 1910.38	Employees designated to assist in emergency evacuation plan	Upon assignment and whenever the plan or the employee's responsibilities under the plan change
	All employees	Upon assignment
Emergency Response/ HAZWOPER 29 CFR 1910.120	HAZWOPER trainers	Maintain academic credentials
	Skilled support personnel	Prior to participation in any emergency response
	Specialists	Annually
	First responders	Initial training before permitted to take part in emergency operations; annual refresher training or demonstration of competency

Standard	Applicability	Frequency
Emergency Response/ HAZWOPER (cont.) 29 CFR 1910.120	Hazardous materials technicians	Initial training before permitted to take part in emergency operations; annual refresher training or demonstration of competency
Ergonomics (voluntary guidelines)	Varies, may include all employees or specific groups	Not specified
Ethylene Oxide 29 CFR 1910.1047	Potentially exposed employees	Upon assignment and annually thereafter
Fire prevention and protection 29 CFR 1910.155	Employees covered by OSHA fire protection standards at 29 CFR 1910	See specific fire protection entries
Fire Brigades 29 CFR 1910.156	Fire brigade members	At least annually, quarterly for those involved in structural firefighting, and frequent enough to ensure safe performance of duties
Fire Extinguishers – Portable 29 CFR 1910.157	All employees except where extinguishers are provided but are not intended for employee use.	Upon assignment and annually thereafter
Fixed Extinguishing Systems 29 CFR 1910.160	Designated employees	Upon assignment and annually thereafter
Fire Detection Systems 29 CFR 1910.164	Designated employees	Upon assignment and refresher training as necessary
Formaldehyde 29 CFR 1910.1048	All employees assigned to workplaces where there is exposure of 0.1 ppm or greater	Upon assignment and whenever a new exposure to formaldehyde is introduced
Glutaraldehyde	Potentially exposed employees	Upon initial assignment and whenever a new hazard is introduced
Hazard Communication 29 CFR 1910.1200	Potentially exposed employees	Upon initial assignment and whenever a new hazard is introduced
Hearing Protection Training Program 29 CFR 1910.95	Employees exposed to over 85db over eight hour TWA	Annually
Laboratory Standard 29 CFR 1910.1450	Employers engaged in the laboratory use of hazardous chemicals	Upon initial assignment and prior to assignments involving new hazards or new exposures; employer is required to determine frequency of refresher information and training

Standard	Applicability	Frequency
Lasers (guidance)	Laser safety officer, qualified and authorized laser operators	Not specified
Laundry/Housekeeping Machinery and Operating Rules 29 CFR 1910.264(d)	Laundry employees	Not specified; also see blood-borne pathogen, hazard communication standards
Lead 29 CFR 1926.62 (construction work) 29 CFR 1910.1025 (general industry)	Employees exposed at or above the action level or where the possibility of skin or eye irritation exists	Upon assignment and annually thereafter
Lockout/Tagout 29 CFR 1910.147	Authorized and affected employees; employees working in areas where lockout/tagout procedures are used	Upon assignment; retraining is required whenever procedures, equipment, or employee's responsibilities change, or employee knowledge is inadequate
Radiation Ionizing 29 CFR 1910.96	Employees working in or frequenting a radiation area	Prior to potential exposure